Neurocognition and Social Cognition in Schizophrenia Patients

Key Issues in Mental Health

Vol. 177

Series Editors

A. Riecher-Rössler Basel
M. Steiner Hamilton

Neurocognition and Social Cognition in Schizophrenia Patients

Basic Concepts and Treatment

Volume Editors

Volker Roder Bern
Alice Medalia New York, N.Y.

16 figures, 1 in color, and 11 tables, 2010

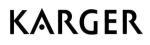

Basel · Freiburg · Paris · London · New York · Bangalore ·
Bangkok · Shanghai · Singapore · Tokyo · Sydney

Key Issues in Mental Health

Formerly published as 'Bibliotheca Psychiatrica' (founded 1917)

Prof. Volker Roder
Head of Therapy Research
University Hospital of Psychiatry
Bern (Switzerland)

Prof. Alice Medalia
Director of Psychiatric
Rehabilitation Services
Columbia University College
of Physicians and Surgeons
New York, N.Y. (USA)

Library of Congress Cataloging-in-Publication Data

Neurocognition and social cognition in schizophrenia patients :
basic concepts and treatment / volume editors, Volker Roder, Alice Medalia.
     p. ; cm. -- (Key issues in mental health, ISSN 1662-4874 ; v. 177)
   Includes bibliographical references and index.
   ISBN 978-3-8055-9338-0 (hard cover : alk . paper)
  1. Schizophrenia--Complications.   2. Cognition disorders.   3.   Cognition.
4. Social perception.   5. Schizophrenics--Rehabilitation.   I.   Roder,
Volker.   II.   Medalia, Alice.   III.   Series: Key issues in mental health, v.
177 . 1662-4874 ;
   [DNLM: 1. Schizophrenia--therapy.   2. Cognition.   3. Cognitive Therapy.
4. Interpersonal Relations.   5. Schizophrenic Psychology.   6.   Social
Adjustment.   W1 BI429 v. 177 2010 / WM 203 N49313 2010]
   RC514 . N4432 2010
   362 . 2'6--dc22
                                    2009047073

Bibliographic Indices. This publication is listed in bibliographic services, including Current Contents® and Index Medicus.

Disclaimer. The statements, opinions and data contained in this publication are solely those of the individual authors and contributors and not of the publisher and the editor(s). The appearance of advertisements in the book is not a warranty, endorsement, or approval of the products or services advertised or of their effectiveness, quality or safety. The publisher and the editor(s) disclaim responsibility for any injury to persons or property resulting from any ideas, methods, instructions or products referred to in the content or advertisements.

Drug Dosage. The authors and the publisher have exerted every effort to ensure that drug selection and dosage set forth in this text are in accord with current recommendations and practice at the time of publication. However, in view of ongoing research, changes in government regulations, and the constant flow of information relating to drug therapy and drug reactions, the reader is urged to check the package insert for each drug for any change in indications and dosage and for added warnings and precautions. This is particularly important when the recommended agent is a new and/or infrequently employed drug.

© Copyright 2010 by S. Karger AG, P.O. Box, CH–4009 Basel (Switzerland)
www.karger.com
Printed in Switzerland on acid-free and non-aging paper (ISO 9706) by Reinhardt Druck, Basel
ISSN 1662–4874
ISBN 978–3–8055–9338–0
eISBN 978–3–8055–9339–7

Contents

Foreword

This book comes at a particularly opportune moment and sets an important corner-stone in this crucial phase of the development of effective cognitive-behavioral treatment strategies for schizophrenia.

If one follows this development over time, the first therapeutic methods mirrored man's picture of himself and assumed a one-sided dependency of behavior on environmental factors. In the 1970s, improving social competence became increasingly important, whereby highly structured programs taught the patient both verbal and non-verbal behavior patterns. It was expected that increased social competence would lead to a better quality of life with deeper social integration. The fact that only moderate therapeutic success was witnessed in this area was seen as a result (among other factors) of the patient's cognitive deficits not being taken into consideration adequately enough. Subsequently, social aspects of the training programs were geared towards overcoming these deficits. As a result, cognitive rehabilitation, which aims to improve the comprehension and processing of information, gained importance. This included both cognitive therapy programs as well as combined cognitive-behavioral approaches. Earlier, cognitive rehabilitation had been neglected for different reasons: cognitive deficits were either considered as epiphenomena, without any functional clinical significance, or as being too deeply rooted in the patient and, thus, not changeable. These assumptions, however, had to be revised when, for example, the lack of learning aptitude postulated for schizophrenic patients was disproved by the complex tasks of tests such as the Wisconsin Card Sorting Test, and the so-called 'vulnerability markers' proved to be modifiable through targeted interventions. Although the initial results for cognitive and, in particular, computer-aided training were encouraging, further investigations only showed limited transfer from such programs to everyday life. The reason for this seemed mainly to be a result of the isolated training of individual cognitive functions, not taking other cognitive deficits and social dimensions into account.

Based on new models of schizophrenia, therefore the combination of elements from cognitive and social therapies appears to be especially promising. On the one hand, mounting evidence suggests that certain neurocognitive and social cognitive deficits are more related to certain areas of functional outcome than psychotic symptoms. The recent advances made in the understanding of these relationships can be directly linked to the development of innovative treatment approaches. On the other hand, the ability to implement the skills practiced in therapy into everyday life requires an implicit knowledge of social situations. In this context, aspects of social perception as well as the perception and management of emotions have gained importance.

Finally, the developments described above have converged with other influences calling for professionals to 'look at the person behind the illness', which appears to find the most visible expression in the concept of recovery. This is the view *Neurocognition and Social Cognition in Schizophrenia Patients: Basic Concepts and Treatment* focuses on; particularly as the editors point out that this book is about much more than just symptomatic relief and stability, but rather the attainment of functional stability and progress in professional formation, work, independent living and social interaction. The understanding and effective treatment of schizophrenia-specific problems with cognition are recognized as central requirements for successful recovery and their various aspects are illuminated: basic information about the nature, measurement and meaning of neurocognitive and social cognitive deficits and processes is provided; the most recent advances in the knowledge about the role of these deficits and processes on functional recovery are highlighted, and the latest innovative approaches to respective treatments, as well as practical examples, are outlined.

Thus, *Neurocognition and Social Cognition in Schizophrenia Patients: Basic Concepts and Treatment* provides a most timely synopsis of this developing field with an emphasis on the integration of neurocognitive and social cognitive functioning in psychiatric rehabilitation. Last but not least, the efforts required to integrate behavior therapy with optimal pharmacotherapy are also acknowledged. From whatever perspective, behavior – cognitive, emotional, social, intellectual and instrumental modes of personal functioning – can be understood as the product of a circular causality between neurophysiological, cognitive, emotional, social and environmental variables constantly interacting with each other. Further advances can only be expected when individual fields within research and practice utilize the current knowledge available in neighboring fields. Overall, this book thus is extremely well suited to scientists and practitioners alike and provides an excellent theoretical and empirical basis for evidence-guided clinical practice as well as for innovative research.

Hans D. Brenner
Valparaiso, December 2009

Preface

People with schizophrenia struggle with an array of positive and negative symptoms, which together often make it difficult to achieve the common life goals of working, living independently, finishing school and forging and maintaining rewarding relationships. The positive symptoms of hallucinations and delusions, disorganization and agitation have received the bulk of attention over the years, and tremendous progress has been made in developing pharmacologic treatments that ameliorate these strikingly abnormal behaviors. With such advances in treatment, more people with schizophrenia live in the community, and the aspiration of achieving recovery is no longer dismissed as impossible but recognized as a meaningful and feasible, although admittedly highly elusive goal.

Why is it that recovery is so difficult to achieve? It is because recovery embraces more than symptomatic relief and stability. Recovery also refers to the attainment of functional stability. Recovered people have made progress in their attempts to finish school, work, live independently and socialize. They are not just living in the community but actively engaged in community life and able to negotiate the challenges with some independence. In the last 2 decades, researchers have carefully studied predictors of functional recovery, and it has become recognized that relief from the positive symptoms is insufficient to garner progress in the functional arena. Rather it is a different array of 'symptoms' that cobble the efforts of patients as they struggle toward recovery; it is the problems with cognition, socialization and motivation.

Impairments in cognition, motivation and socialization have been recognized as core features of schizophrenia for over 100 years. At the turn of the 20th century Emil Kraeplin wrote about a progressive decline in the cognitive abilities of attention, problem solving and learning, which he speculated was negatively effecting social, vocational and independent functioning. Since he identified the problems, numerous studies have been and continue to be done to characterize the nature of the deficits. When the role of these deficits in functional outcome had been demonstrated, the clinical significance of developing treatments for these disabilities gained recognition.

Cognition is a term that broadly refers to thinking abilities. It encompasses the range of skills from isolated processes like memory and attention, which are the focus of neuropsychological investigations and therapies, to the form and content of thought, which are often the focus of cognitive behavioral therapies. The study of cognitive processes appreciates that while most processes are neuropsychological, some are primarily in the service of social interactions, and the term social cognition is used to identify those particular processes. The cognitive ability to perceive, interpret and generate responses to social interactions is included in the term social cognition. Together neurocognition and social cognition refer to the basic processes that allow one to learn about, understand and know the world one lives in.

This edited volume addresses the neurocognitive and social cognitive processes that are known to be disrupted in schizophrenia. The focus on these disorders appreciates that they are a key determinant of functional recovery and that to change functionally often requires that neurocognition and social cognition be addressed. The volume is intended to provide practicing clinicians, emerging schizophrenia researchers and students of psychotic disorders with the latest information about the neurocognitive and social cognitive deficits in schizophrenia. This way professionals working with persons with schizophrenia will have the knowledge and tools they need to develop and provide competent professional care.

This volume is organized to provide information about the characterization of neurocognitive and social cognitive deficits as well as treatment approaches which target these symptoms. We invited leading experts – physicians and psychologists – from Europe and the USA to present the 'state of the art' in the different fields. To start, chapter 1, by Robert S. Kern and William P. Horan, defines what is meant by these terms and reviews the methods of measurement that are used in different clinical and research settings. Chapter 2, by John S. Brekke and Eri Nakagami, explains why neurocognition and social cognition are relevant to functional recovery and reviews the literature which delineated the ways that these deficits impact work, social and educational outcomes. Given the sobering results on functional outcome when treatments only focus on positive symptoms, there is a growing interest in alternative treatments that target neurocognitive and social cognitive deficits. Chapter 3, by Matthew M. Kurtz and Gudrun Sartory, provides an overview of the behavioral approaches to treating neurocognition. The subchapter by Elizabeth W. Twamley, Cynthia H. Zurhellen and Lea Vella describes a concrete therapy approach for neurocognition, while chapter 4, by Wolfgang Wölwer, Dennis R. Combs, Nicole Frommann and David L. Penn, synthesizes the literature on behavioral treatments of social cognitive deficits. The subchapter by Roland Vauth provides an example of a treatment approach which was designed to train social cognition and thereby enhance emotional intelligence. Chapter 5 by Volker Roder, Lea Hulka and Alice

Medalia gives an overview of treatments integrating neurocognition and social cognition (and partly social skills). Two subchapters illustrate examples for these integrative approaches: Alice Medalia and Elisa Mambrino present the Neuropsychological and Educational Approach to Remediation (NEAR); Daniel R. Müller and Volker Roder describe the Integrated Psychological Therapy (IPT) and the Integrated Neurocognitive Therapy (INT) with concrete guidelines for their application. The pharmacologic treatment of cognition is a burgeoning area, and chapter 6, by Alex Hofer and W. Wolfgang Fleischhacker, reviews the various approaches that are being taken to drug development. Finally, because amotivation is a core feature of schizophrenia and impacts not only the functional outcome but also the ability to engage and benefit from therapies, chapter 7, by Alice Medalia and Jimmy Choi, considers the relevance of motivational theories for understanding how to maximize benefit from therapies that provide cognitive enhancement.

With the interest in promoting functional recovery in schizophrenia comes the need for clinicians and researchers to understand the issues that hamper a successful outcome. Treating symptoms is not enough – the overall goal of any intervention is to help a person integrate and function adaptively in society. This collection of chapters usefully characterizes the nature of the neurocognitive and social cognitive deficits known to negatively impact the functional outcome, as well as the efforts underway to treat them. The terminology, measurement strategies and therapeutic approaches are thoughtfully considered and reviewed. We would like to express gratitude to the authors for contributing to this volume and to Professor Anita Riecher (University Hospital of Psychiatry, Basel, Switzerland) for her vision in choosing this as a topic of interest. It is hoped that these chapters will promote discussion, more research and the further development and improvement of interventions for people with schizophrenia.

Alice Medalia
Volker Roder
New York and Bern, August 2009

Roder V, Medalia A (eds): Neurocognition and Social Cognition in Schizophrenia Patients. Basic Concepts and Treatment. Key Issues Ment Health. Basel, Karger, 2010, vol 177, pp 1–22

1

Definition and Measurement of Neurocognition and Social Cognition

Robert S. Kern[a,b] · William P. Horan[a,b]

[a]Department of Psychiatry and Biobehavioral Sciences, David Geffen School of Medicine at UCLA, and [b]Department of Veterans Affairs VISN 22 Mental Illness Research, Education and Clinical Center, Los Angeles, Calif., USA

Abstract

Disturbances in neurocognition and social cognition are widely recognized as core features of schizophrenia. In this chapter, we provide a critical review of measurement in these 2 areas. For neurocognition, we compare 3 approaches: (a) hybrid batteries, (b) computer-based batteries and (c) the MATRICS Consensus Cognitive Battery. For social cognition, we compare measures used to assess 5 key domains: (a) emotional processing, (b) social perception, (c) social knowledge, (d) attribution bias and (e) theory of mind. We conclude with a section on the promise of developing new treatments in neurocognition and social cognition that will rely, in part, on the advances in measurement within these areas.   Copyright © 2010 S. Karger AG, Basel

In this chapter we define neurocognition and social cognition, and review methods of measurement in these 2 areas in schizophrenia. The first section on neurocognition will describe and contrast 3 types of neurocognitive batteries: (a) hybrid batteries, (b) computer-based neurocognitive batteries and (c) the MATRICS Consensus Cognitive Battery (MCCB). The second section on social cognition will describe measures commonly used to assess 5 domains within this construct: (a) emotional processing, (b) social perception, (c) social knowledge, (d) attributional bias and (e) theory of mind. We conclude with a section on the promise of developing new treatments for neurocognitive and social cognitive deficits as a means of improving functioning in persons with schizophrenia.

Neurocognition in Schizophrenia

Definition of Neurocognition

The clinical observation that neurocognitive impairment was a primary feature of schizophrenia can be traced back to the early writings of Emil Kraepelin [1] at the turn of the 20th century and his use of the term 'dementia praecox' to describe the disorder. He noted that the onset typically occurred in early adulthood (praecox) and resulted in progressive functional and intellectual decline (dementia) in most cases. In his writings on the clinical presentation of dementia praecox, Kraepelin described a wide range of neurocognitive impairments that included disturbances in attention, learning and problem-solving. These disturbances were noted to have marked effects on social behavior, independent living and work functioning.

A general definition provides that neurocognition can be thought of as encompassing all aspects of learning about, understanding and knowing the world around oneself [2]. It includes all of one's mental abilities, such as attention, perception, memory, language processing, visuospatial ability, executive functions and others used to interact with and make sense of the environment. In schizophrenia research, 7 separable neurocognitive areas have been identified as being of primary interest: attention/vigilance, speed of processing, working memory, verbal learning, visual learning, reasoning and problem-solving as well as social cognition [3]. Of these, social cognition appears to hold a unique place in understanding functioning and will be discussed separately within this chapter.

Neurocognition as a Core Deficit of Schizophrenia

It is widely held that neurocognitive deficits represent a core feature of schizophrenia [4]. That is, they reflect a primary deficit and are not secondary to other features of the illness (clinical symptoms) or treatment-related factors (medication effects) and are common to most, if not all, persons with schizophrenia [2]. For example, a report based on a large, diverse sample indicated that approximately 90% of the persons with schizophrenia show clinically significant levels of impairment in at least 1 neurocognitive domain and 75% show impairment in at least 2 [5]. These figures are probably underestimates when one considers the likelihood that a number of individuals who go on to develop schizophrenia had higher than average premorbid levels of neurocognitive functioning.

Schizophrenia is typically characterized as a disorder with generalized neurocognitive dysfunction that includes specific domains that are more adversely affected than others [6–8]. In chronic, stable outpatient samples, clinically meaningful differences are found between patients and healthy controls across a wide range of neurocognitive domains with effect sizes typically ranging between 0.75 and 1.5 [6]. In the context of these generalized deficits, converging evidence from independent reports and meta-analyses indicates that the impairments to 1 aspect of memory functioning (i.e. learning), commonly measured using list learning tasks, are more severely affected than other areas of neurocognition [6, 7]. The level of neurocognitive impairment remains relatively stable during the adult years (ages 21–55), and persists into late life, when there may be further decline.

Importantly, neurocognitive deficits appear to be relatively independent of the clinical symptoms of the disorder. Although it is somewhat intuitive to expect neurocognitive functioning to be adversely affected by positive symptoms of psychosis (e.g. hallucinations, delusions), there is little evidence to support such a relationship [8–11]. Neurocognitive deficits show a stronger, more consistent relationship with disorganized and negative symptoms (e.g. avolition, alogia, apathy, anhedonia) [12, 13], but the amount of shared variance remains relatively small (5–10%). The relative independence between neurocognitive functioning and clinical symptoms is further supported by data from studies that reveal the persistence of neurocognitive impairments in both psychotic and remitted states [14]. Also, deficits occur in prodromal samples and meta-analyses of family studies of 'at-risk children and adolescents' [15].

The scope and severity of neurocognitive deficits seen in persons with schizophrenia do not appear to be secondary to treatment with antipsychotic medications. In general, second-generation antipsychotic medications are not associated with negative effects on neurocognition and may, in fact, convey modest neurocognitive benefits compared to conventional agents [16–19]. It is not clear, however, whether the observed differences are due to the dose levels of conventional agents used in many studies or a reduction in extrapyramidal symptoms and concomitant administration of anticholinergic agents associated with the treatment of second-generation agents [20].

Evidence indicates that the neurocognitive functioning of individuals with schizophrenia is intimately related to real-world functioning. Three reviews of the literature [21–23] show cross-sectional and prospective ties between selected areas of neurocognitive functioning and areas of functional outcome, including community functioning (e.g. broader aspects of work and social functioning), ability to perform instrumental role skills and psychosocial rehabilitation success. For individual cognitive domains, the findings for memory functioning, and verbal learning in particular, appear especially robust [22]. Though more modest degrees of variance are explained at the individual domain level, the amount can be quite large when the effects of neurocognitive functioning are considered more broadly. For example, when multiple neurocognitive domains are included in a summary score, as much as 30% of the variance in functional outcome can be explained [22].

In sum, neurocognitive deficits are seen in most, if not all, persons with schizophrenia, they are relatively independent of psychiatric symptoms and drug effects, and are related to real-world functioning.

Measurement of Neurocognition

The measurement of neurocognition can be carved up in a number of ways. We opted to cover 3 methods that are widely used and provide contrast: (a) hybrid batteries,

(b) computer-based batteries and (c) the MCCB [24]. The MCCB used a consensus-based approach to address the shortcomings of other neurocognitive assessment batteries. The following sections describe and critically evaluate these 3 approaches.

Hybrid Batteries

Hybrid batteries are comprised of a number of different neurocognitive tests with the aim of covering a broad range of neurocognitive domains. The number of domains covered by the battery and the number of tests within each domain are controlled by the investigator and are free to vary across studies. The origins of the hybrid battery can likely be traced to the Halstead-Reitan neuropsychological battery [25], which used a variety of different tests to assess selected neurocognitive domains in the assessment of persons with traumatic brain injury and other neurocognitive disorders (e.g., Alzheimer's disease). In the assessment of persons with schizophrenia, tests from the Halstead-Reitan battery continue to be widely used (e.g. Trail Making Test [26], Wisconsin Card Sorting Test [27]). Results from hybrid batteries have been the primary source of data for meta-analyses of neurocognitive studies of schizophrenia described in the previous section [6]. When examining group means, persons with schizophrenia typically fall within the 2nd to 15th percentiles on tests from representative hybrid batteries [28]. A large number of studies confirm severe deficits to verbal learning ability, executive functioning and attention/vigilance with milder deficits to language-based skills such as vocabulary and naming ability. Depending on the nature of the sample (e.g. chronic inpatients), the magnitude of impairment can be quite high (2–5 standard deviations below the mean of norms for adults of comparable demographic make-up). Though typically comprised of paper-and-pencil measures, hybrid batteries may include computer-based tests for the assessment of selected constructs (e.g. attention/vigilance).

It should be noted that 2 standardized paper-and-pencil test batteries developed for use in schizophrenia, the Repeatable Battery for the Assessment of Neuropsychological Status and Brief Assessment of Cognition in Schizophrenia, grew out of this literature [29, 30]. These are brief batteries (approximately 30 min in length) that assess a subset of neurocognitive domains. They show patient versus control differences comparable with larger batteries with effect sizes that range from approximately 0.8 to 1.5 for the Brief Assessment of Cognition in Schizophrenia [31] to approximately 1.0–2.0 for the Repeatable Battery for the Assessment of Neuropsychological Status [30]. Their psychometric properties however, such as test-retest reliability, indicate that they tend to perform better as an overall composite index of neurocognitive functioning than at the domain level.

The primary advantage of hybrid batteries is their familiarity to both researchers and clinicians. Tests commonly included within these batteries (e.g. executive functioning tests such as the Wisconsin Card Sorting Test [27], list learning and delayed recall and recognition tests, verbal fluency tests, digit span tests, symbol digit substitution type tests, psychomotor tests) are widely used in clinical and research environments and therefore facilitate the interpretation of findings to a broad audience. Another advantage of hybrid batteries is their flexibility. The number of domains and the number of tests within a domain can be adjusted to suit the needs of the assessment or focus of research. For example, a study investigating the acute effects of an experimental drug on memory functioning may wish to expand the number of measures included in this domain to help ensure that the construct is adequately captured by the battery.

However, hybrid batteries are subject to a number of criticisms, most of which are attributable to the absence of standardization in the configuration of tests and the selection of dependent measures within these batteries. First, there is no consensus about categorization of tests by neurocognitive domain. For example, tests like verbal fluency (e.g. FAS) are sometimes listed under different neurocognitive domains (e.g. semantic memory, speed of processing or language functioning) depending on the individual study, thus leaving the findings ambiguous as to which area of neurocognition is measured. Second, there are inconsistencies in the selection of dependent measures used in tests that yield more than a single index of performance. For example, many tests within the domains of attention, memory and executive functioning include multiple performance measures leaving the selection up to the investigator. The absence of standardization in the selection of dependent measures compromises the interpretation of findings across studies.

There are other more subtle disadvantages as well. First, some studies use principle component analyses or factor-analytic methods to reduce the number of variables and limit the risk of type I error [32]. Though advantageous in attaining variable reduction, factor scores are dependent on a study's sample characteristics and are inherently difficult to replicate. Second, the test order is not standardized across studies. The administration order can adversely affect the performance on certain tests within a battery. Most frequently observed problems of this type occur when tests that require similar processing demands are administered adjacent to one another. For example, the administration of multiple memory tests or ones with high language processing demands may produce interference effects that adversely affect the performance on later-occurring tests within a series. Finally, there is a risk for uncontrolled effects of fatigue in batteries that are not standardized and vary considerably in length and processing demands. In sum, despite the popularity of hybrid batteries, the absence of standardization poses substantial concern for impacts on performance and limits the interpretation of findings across studies.

Computer-Based Batteries

Computer-based neurocognitive batteries have become increasingly popular as evidenced by the ever-growing number of batteries developed over the past 10–15 years (Cambridge Automated Neuropsychological Test Battery [33, 34], MicroCog [35], Neurobehavioral Evaluation System [36], WebNeuro [37], Penn computerized neuropsychological battery [38, 39], IntegNeuro [40], CogState [41], Cogtest [42], Mindstreams [43], Computerized Multiphasic Interactive Neurocognitive Dual

Display [44]). Like paper-and-pencil hybrid batteries, these assess a range of neurocognitive functions and can be administered by trained research or clinical staff under appropriate supervision. In general, these batteries do not require specialized software or technical expertise to administer and score, and they can be installed on desktop or laptop computers. At present, there are no meta-analyses of these batteries in studies with schizophrenia patients, and data for some of the newer batteries are particularly sparse. From the available data, patients show differences from controls across the vast majority of neurocognitive domains with deficits in attention, memory, and executive functioning noted as severest [34, 40, 43, 45, 46]. The magnitude of impairment appears roughly comparable to that seen on paper-and-pencil tests measuring the equivalent construct [39, 46].

In the American Psychological Association's 1986 guidelines for use and interpretation of computerized tests to assess neurocognition, a number of specific advantages over paper-and-pencil tests were cited [47]. Among these were: (a) administration and scoring of individual tests within each battery is automated, thus standardizing these procedures, reducing human error and facilitating replicability across studies using the same battery; (b) computer-based batteries allow greater precision on tests that involve measurement of reaction time or require precision in stimulus presentation (e.g. exposure time, between-stimulus intervals, etc.); (c) scored data are saved in files on the computer, thus facilitating the protection and security of collected data, and (d) many of these batteries include their own normative data and yield individual test scores that can be compared directly with one another using a common reference sample and a standard scale of measurement to facilitate interpretation.

The limitations associated with computer-based batteries include questionable support for the construct validity of certain measures, the narrowness in range of constructs covered in some batteries (heavy reliance on motor and visuospatial tasks), difficulties in adapting some tests to computer administration, and problems with lost or irretrievable data. Though many paper-and-pencil neurocognitive tests have been examined in factor-analytic studies conducted by independent investigators [3], fewer computer-based batteries have gone through similar methods to provide support that the individual tests included in these batteries are measuring the construct of interest [48]. With respect to computer administration, although there are advantages for measuring neurocognitive domains such as attention/vigilance via computerized continuous performance tests, there are greater difficulties adapting computerized tests to measures that require fine motor drawing skills such as visual learning tests. Finally, despite the advantages associated with automated scoring and saving scored data files, computer-based tests are frequently noted to be the ones most often associated with missing data in clinical trials.

MATRICS Consensus Cognitive Battery
The MATRICS process has been explained in detail elsewhere [49–51]. Briefly, we describe the 10 steps that went into the development of the MCCB (see fig. 1).

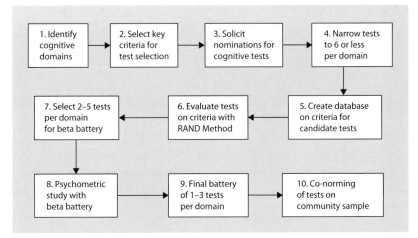

Fig. 1. Steps in the development of the MCCB. Adapted from Green et al. [49].

Initially, experts from various areas (e.g. cognitive deficits in schizophrenia, clinical neuropsychology, clinical trial methodology) were invited to participate in a structured phone interview survey. The results of the survey in conjunction with review of data from 16 factor-analytic studies of neurocognition in schizophrenia were presented and discussed at an in-person meeting. Following the meeting, the MATRICS Neurocognition Committee met and agreed upon 7 separable neurocognitive domains that were key to the assessment of persons with schizophrenia (see table 1) as well as selection criteria to use in evaluating nominated tests. The selection criteria included: (a) test-retest reliability, (b) utility as a repeated measure, (c) relationship with functional outcome, and (d) practicality and tolerability.

Over 90 tests were initially nominated. This group was narrowed down to 36 for consideration and review by a RAND Panel of Experts. A database that contained data from published and unpublished studies on the selection criteria for each of the 36 tests was created by MATRICS staff. The RAND Panel reviewed the database, made ratings on the 4 selection criteria for each test and discussed discrepancies between panelists at an in-person meeting. The results of the RAND Panel were reviewed and discussed by the MATRICS Neurocognition Committee, which led to the formulation of the β-version of the battery (20 tests across 7 neurocognitive domains). The β-version of the battery was then evaluated in a prospective study of 176 schizophrenia and schizoaffective disorder outpatients at 5 participating sites in the USA (Duke University, Harvard University, University of Kansas, University of Maryland and University of California, Los Angeles). The results from the study were reviewed by the MATRICS Neurocognition Committee and led to the selection of 10 tests for inclusion in the final MATRICS battery. The final MATRICS battery was then co-normed in a sample of 300 community residents drawn from the same 5 research

Table 1. Seven neurocognitive domains assessed by the MCCB

Neurocognitive domain	MCCB test
Attention/vigilance	Continuous Performance Test – Identical Pairs version [140, 141]
Speed of processing	Trail Making Test – Part A [26] Brief Assessment of Cognition in Schizophrenia: Symbol Coding subtest [29] Category fluency – animal naming [142, 143]
Working memory	Letter-Number Span [143] Wechsler Memory Scale – III: Spatial Span subtest [144]
Verbal learning	Hopkins Verbal Learning Test – Revised [145]
Visual learning	Brief Visuospatial Memory Test – Revised [146]
Reasoning and problem solving	Neuropsychological Assessment Battery: Mazes subtest [147]
Social cognition	Mayer-Salovey-Caruso Emotional Intelligence Test: Managing Emotions [74]

sites and the data used to develop a scoring program that provided standard scores (T scores with a mean of 50 and standard deviation of 10) for each of the 10 tests and 7 neurocognitive domains.

The MATRICS battery became available for distribution in April 2006. Two published reports on the MATRICS battery from a young, adolescent schizophrenia spectrum disorder sample and a chronic schizophrenia/schizoaffective disorder sample, respectively, show a relatively similar pattern of results [46, 52]. The magnitude of impairment in the adolescent sample yielded effect sizes that ranged from 0.8 to 1.8 across neurocognitive domains (with the curious exception of social cognition); the chronic sample yielded similar results with effect sizes ranging from approximately 0.75 to 1.5 across individual tests.

The advantages of the MATRICS battery include the ability to directly compare findings across studies using standardized scores with demographic correction derived from a common normative sample. Many of the limitations associated with the hybrid batteries and absence of standardization of tests and dependent measures are addressed in a consensus-based battery. There are no problems with inconsistencies in the selection of neurocognitive domains, tests, order of administration or selection of dependent variables that impede interpretation across studies. A disadvantage of the MATRICS battery is the narrow selection of measures within neurocognitive domains. Five of the 7 neurocognitive domains are assessed by a single test. Hence, the interpretation of findings largely rests on the ability of that particular test to adequately capture that particular cognitive construct. To this end, supplemental tests that could be added to the MATRICS battery to supplement memory and reasoning as well as problem-solving domains were recommended.

In sum, despite specific advantages of hybrid and computer-based neurocognitive batteries in the assessment of neurocognition in persons with schizophrenia, both approaches have noteworthy limitations. The MCCB also has acknowledged limitations but has a key advantage in being consensus-based, which promotes its acceptance as a standard for the field. We now transition to the examination of measurement within social cognition, an area that holds a unique role in amplifying our understanding of the cognitive processes involved in the social functioning of persons with schizophrenia.

Social Cognition

In the next section, we define social cognition and review existing measures that assess the different subareas of social cognition.

Definition of Social Cognition

Social cognition is a multifaceted construct that broadly refers to the mental operations underlying social interactions. It has been defined as 'the ability to construct representations of the relations between oneself and others, and to use those representations flexibly to guide social behavior' [53]. Social cognitive operations typically include perceiving, interpreting and generating responses to the emotions, intentions and dispositions of others [54–56]. Simply put, social cognition is a set of skills that people use to understand and effectively interact with other people. Therefore, problems in social cognition, such as misperceptions and unexpected reactions to and from other people, can be expected to adversely impact functioning across a variety of domains. Basic behavioral and neuroscience research in the field of social cognition has burgeoned over the past decade [57, 58], providing a rich theoretical and methodological foundation to investigate social cognitive disturbances in neuropsychiatric disorders such as a schizophrenia.

Social cognition in schizophrenia is a rapidly growing research area, as reflected in an online search of PsycINFO for the key words 'social cognition' combined with schizophrenia (see fig. 2). As can be readily seen, the number of studies referencing these terms has increased dramatically over the past 5 years. As an indication of social cognition's increasing visibility, the investigators of the NIMH-MATRICS identified it as 1 of 7 key cognitive domains that should be routinely assessed in clinical trials of new cognitive enhancers for schizophrenia [3]. This section of the chapter provides a brief overview of the major domains of social cognition studied in schizophrenia and the types of measures commonly used to assess them.

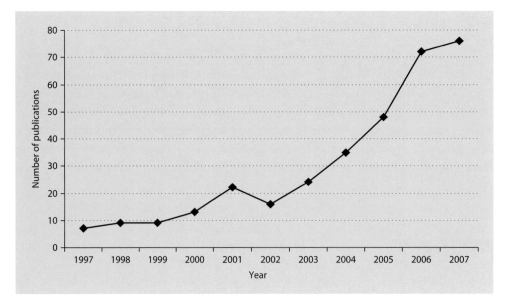

Fig. 2. Number of publications in social cognition and schizophrenia by year. Reproduced from Green et al. [59].

Domains of Social Cognition Studied in Schizophrenia

The rapid expansion of social cognition research in schizophrenia has resulted in the use of an increasingly diverse range of terminology and assessment techniques. In light of the diverse range of terms and paradigms used across studies, the NIMH recently sponsored a consensus-building workshop to integrate research in this area and guide future research efforts [59]. This section is organized in terms of the 5 broad domains of social cognition suggested by this work group. We describe the key social cognitive processes subsumed within each domain and critically evaluate commonly used assessment techniques, which are summarized in table 2.

Emotional Processing
Emotional processing broadly refers to aspects of perceiving and using emotion to facilitate adaptive functioning. One influential model of emotional processing defines 'emotional intelligence' as a set of skills that combines emotions and cognition. The model is comprised of 4 emotional processing components, including identifying, facilitating, understanding and managing emotions [60, 61].

Affect perception, which falls in the identifying emotions component of this model, has been the most extensively studied social cognitive process in schizophrenia. Deficits have been most frequently documented in paradigms that require subjects to identify or discriminate between emotions displayed in still photographs of

Table 2. Domains of social cognition assessed in schizophrenia

Domain	Representative tasks
Emotional processing	Facial Emotion Identification Test [148] Voice Emotion Identification Test [148] Penn Computerized Neurocognitive Battery – Emotion Recognition Test [70] The Awareness of Social Inference Test – Part 1 [72] Mayer-Salovey-Caruso Emotional Intelligence Test [74]
Social perception	Profile of Non-Verbal Sensitivity [82] Social Cue Recognition Test [80]
Social knowledge	Situational Features Recognition Test [93] Schema Comprehension Sequencing Test-Revised [94]
Attributional bias	Attributional Style Questionnaire [101] Internal, Personal and Situational Attributions Questionnaire [97] Ambiguous Intentions Hostility Questionnaire [103]
Theory of Mind	False belief stories [108] False belief picture sequencing [111] Hinting task [109] Reading the Mind in the Eyes test [110] The Awareness of Social Inferences Test – Parts 2 and 3 [72]

a single person's face. Similar problems are found in studies of perceiving emotion in vocalizations or videotaped monologues, with deficits sometimes found to be severer for certain negative (fear, disgust) compared to positive emotions. The magnitude of patient versus control differences is large; a recent meta-analysis of 86 studies using diverse tasks reported an overall effect size of –0.91 [62]. These deficits appear to be present from early in the course of schizophrenia, relatively stable over time and detectable in high-risk subjects [63–66].

The limitations of commonly used affect perception tasks include their psycho-metric properties, which are often found to be less than optimal [63, 67, 68], and an ongoing debate about whether affect perception problems in schizophrenia reflect a specific deficit or part of a general cognitive deficit [69]. Questions have also been raised about whether viewing still pictures of faces or listening to tape-recorded voices adequately captures the complexity of affect perception abilities required for successful social interactions [68], though tasks with better psychometrics [70] and that use dynamic stimuli are increasingly available [71, 72]. Despite these limitations, deficits on affect perception tasks show clear functional relevance for schizophrenia, as they are consistently related to various aspects of social competence and function-ing [73].

Other aspects of emotion processing have been much less extensively studied, and the measures used vary widely. For example, the social cognitive measure included in the MCCB, the managing emotions subtest of the Mayer-Salovey-Caruso Emotional Intelligence Test [74], involves reading brief social/emotional vignettes and responding to questions about how individuals manage, regulate or facilitate emotion in themselves and others. Deficits on the managing emotions and the other performance-based Mayer-Salovey-Caruso Emotional Intelligence Test subtests have been documented in schizophrenia [75, 76]. Patients have also shown abnormalities on various self-report measures of emotional processing and on experimental paradigms that assess how patients regulate (e.g. intentionally suppress, reappraise) their responses to evocative stimuli [77–79].

Social Perception

Social perception refers to a person's ability to judge social cues from contextual information and communicative gestures, including awareness of the roles, rules and goals that typically characterize social situations and guide social interactions [80, 81]. In social perception tasks, participants must process nonverbal, paraverbal and/or verbal cues to make inferences about complex or ambiguous social situations. Individuals may be asked to identify interpersonal features in a situation such as intimacy, status, mood state and veracity.

The most commonly used tasks in this domain were developed nearly 20 years ago. For example, the Profile of Nonverbal Sensitivity [82] involves watching 2-second videos of a Caucasian woman that include facial expressions, vocal intonations and/or body gestures, and selecting from 2 labels (e.g. saying a prayer, talking to a lost child) the one that best described the most likely context for the social cue(s). Similarly, the Social Cue Recognition Test [80] involves watching videotaped vignettes of 2–3 actors engaged in low-emotion (e.g. 2 friends assembling a puzzle) or high-emotion (e.g. a husband and wife fighting about their children) situations, and answering true-false questions about concrete and abstract cues displayed during the interactions. A number of studies document performance deficits on these types of task in people with schizophrenia at various stages of illness [80, 83–85] as well as in their unaffected relatives [86].

A handful of studies using more contemporary stimuli have assessed the impact of contextual information on social perception in schizophrenia. For example, a series of studies by Green and colleagues used paradigms in which subjects evaluate the emotions or mental states of people shown in pictures either in isolation (i.e. no social context) or embedded in a surrounding social context. Schizophrenia patients' socioemotional judgments were significantly less influenced by contextual information than those of healthy controls [87, 88]. Along these lines, a few other research groups have reported deficits in extracting information from complex emotional scenes, and orienting to and visual scanning of social contextual information in schizophrenia [89, 90]. These skills required to successfully perform social perception tasks rely on subjects' knowledge about the rules that typically govern social situations, which overlaps with the following domain.

Social Knowledge

This area refers to awareness of the roles, rules and goals that characterize social situations and guide social interactions [81, 91, 92]. Social knowledge (also called social schema) can be measured with paper-and-pencil tests that assess one's awareness of what is socially expected in different situations (e.g. in a doctor's office versus in a restaurant). It has been studied somewhat less than the other areas in schizophrenia, and it overlaps with social perception; successful social knowledge requires awareness of which cues occur typically in specific social situations (i.e. social perception) and how one is supposed to respond to them.

As with social perception, the most common instruments used to measure this domain were developed nearly 20 years ago, primarily assessing awareness of what is socially expected in different situations. For example, compared to controls, schizophrenia patients have shown impairment on the Social Features Recognition Test [93], a multiple-choice test that assesses participants' knowledge of the characteristics (e.g. roles, rules) of different social situations. Similarly, impairments have been found on the Schema Comprehension Sequencing Test-Revised [94, 95], which requires subjects to sort index cards describing actions into meaningful sequences of social behavior. A limitation of these tasks is that they are rather simple, often resulting in ceiling effects in studies of schizophrenia [e.g. 92, 95]. Despite the measurement limitations, social knowledge appears to be an important construct and is commonly viewed as an initial step and prerequisite for adequate social perception and competence [96]. In addition, performance on tasks measuring both social perception and social knowledge has demonstrated relations to various aspects of social functioning in over 10 studies [73].

Attributional Bias

Attributional style refers to how individuals characteristically explain the causes for positive and negative events in their lives. Attributions can be measured by questionnaires [97] or rated from transcripts of interactions [98]. In research involving both psychiatric and nonpsychiatric samples, key distinctions are typically made between external personal attributions (i.e. causes attributed to other people), external situational attributions (i.e. causes attributed to situational factors) and internal attributions (i.e. causes due to oneself).

In schizophrenia research, this aspect of social cognition has been studied primarily in the context of understanding the psychological mechanisms of persecutory delusions and paranoid beliefs. For example, individuals with persecutory delusions may tend to blame others rather than situations for negative events, an attributional style known as a 'personalizing bias' [99, 100]. Individuals characterized by this style may also be prone to attribute ambiguous events to hostile intentions of others or to jump quickly to conclusions when forming opinions about others without modifying their impressions based on contextual information. Instrumentation in this area is limited, and the results have been somewhat mixed. However, associations between paranoid beliefs and attributional style have been found using socioemotional information processing tasks and self-report measures, such as the Attributional Style Questionnaire [101] or the Internal, Personal and Situational Attributions Questionnaire [97, 102], which describes various hypothetical situations and asks participants to generate explanations for why the events occurred.

Existing measures have been criticized as having poor psychometric properties and questionable external validity [100, 102]. A recently developed self-report measure, the Ambiguous Intentions Hostility Questionnaire [103], and alternative systems for coding attributions from narrative provided by subjects [104, 105], may help address these issues. It also remains unclear whether disturbances in attributional bias are best viewed as state-like phenomena related to certain psychotic symptoms or an enduring, trait-like deficit. Finally, despite some encouraging initial evidence [73], the links between attributional biases and functional outcome in schizophrenia remain largely unexplored.

Theory of Mind

The Theory of Mind (also called mental state attribution or mentalizing) typically involves the ability to infer intentions, dispositions and beliefs of others [106, 107]. Processes typically associated with the Theory of Mind involve the ability to understand false beliefs, hints, intentions, humor, deceptions, metaphor and irony. Theory of Mind studies in schizophrenia have relied heavily on paper-and-pencil measures, such as short stories or sequential picture sets of line drawings [108–112], several of which were passed down from the developmental literature examining the social development of healthy children and those with autism spectrum disorders. For example, false belief tasks involve reading short stories and answering questions to assess whether individuals are capable of understanding basic first-order false beliefs (i.e. that someone can hold a false belief about a state of the world) or more complex second-order false beliefs (i.e. that someone can have a false belief about the belief of another person). Other paradigms evaluate whether subjects can arrange cartoon panels in a coherent fashion by using knowledge about the complex mental states (e.g. intention to deceive) of the characters depicted in the pictures [113].

Schizophrenia patients consistently show deficits on a variety of tasks believed to involve abilities related to the Theory of Mind [114, 115], with meta-analyses reporting overall effect sizes based on over 30 studies ranging from 0.90 to 1.25 [116, 117]. Although performance seems to be particularly impaired in acutely symptomatic patients, substantial deficits are also found in remitted patients [116]. In addition, these deficits are present throughout the course of illness and detectable in high-risk subjects [116, 118, 119]. Initial studies support linkages between the Theory of

Mind and functioning in schizophrenia [73], although these relations have only been addressed in a handful of studies.

Many of the measures used in this area are not ideally suited for adults with schizophrenia because they were developed for children and are consequently prone to ceiling effects, demonstrate poor reliability [e.g. 120], or place strong demands on reading, comprehension and working memory abilities. In addition, paper-and-pencil measures do not capture dynamic characteristics that convey meaning in daily social interactions. Some more developmentally appropriate and alternative paradigms have recently been applied to schizophrenia. For example, patients have been found to show deficits on the Awareness of Social Inferences Test (part 3; [72]), a paradigm specifically developed for adults that assesses mentalizing processes depicted in videotaped interactions between adults, such as forming inferences about others' intentions and beliefs, as well as detecting sarcasm and white lies [121]. Another recent study found mentalizing impairment in schizophrenia using a computerized paradigm derived from social psychology that depicts dynamic 'interactions' among animated figures [122]. These dynamic types of paradigms may more directly assess processes related to the Theory of Mind processes required for effective everyday interactions.

In summary, it is increasingly clear that many people with schizophrenia show substantial impairments across multiple domains of social cognition. In several domains, these appear to be enduring deficits that show meaningful links to social functioning. While the categories identified above provide a reasonable structure for organizing social cognition research in schizophrenia, it should be noted that the boundaries between these categories are not absolute and that there is considerable overlap among them. As discussed further below, our understanding of the key social cognitive deficits involved in schizophrenia and refinement of the methods used to assess them will benefit from ongoing developments in basic social and affective neuroscience. Nonetheless, the available evidence base has led to a great deal of interest in the possibility of intervening at the level of social cognition as a means of improving social outcome.

Neurocognition and Social Cognition as Treatment Targets

The consideration of neurocognition as a treatment target has developed in part due to the growing awareness that clinical treatments that target solely psychiatric symptoms have done little to promote functional recovery, a finding that extends back over 100 years [123]. In a storied history dating back to 1900 that has included efforts with convulsive therapy, frontal lobotomies, neuroleptic medications and second-generation antipsychotic agents, there has been relatively little movement in returning persons with schizophrenia back to work or improving the quality of their social lives. The employment rates continue close to 10–15% [124], and large numbers are homeless, unmarried and have few close friends [125, 126]. Given these sobering results, the time is ripe to consider an alternative target that might yield greater effects on functional outcome. As noted earlier in this chapter, neurocognitive deficits are now widely recognized as a core feature of the disorder, affecting the vast majority of persons with schizophrenia. They are present at the onset of the illness, persist throughout the adult lifespan, and are related to community functioning. Hence, there is wide recognition that the development of treatments to address the neurocognitive deficits of schizophrenia is a worthwhile endeavor [50].

Enthusiasm about intervening at the level of social cognition has been bolstered by 3 lines of evidence. First, as described above, deficits on social cognitive tasks are related to various aspects of social competence and functioning [73]. Second, there is a general consensus that social cognition is distinct from, though related to, basic neurocognition and other clinical features of schizophrenia [127–130]. Along these lines, functional neuroimaging research increasingly suggests that the processing of social and nonsocial stimuli relies on semi-independent neural systems for processing social and nonsocial stimuli [58, 131, 132], and dissociations between social and nonsocial cognition are evident in various clinical conditions [133–135]. Third, recent studies suggest that social cognition shows *unique* relationships to functional outcome, above and beyond basic cognition [73]. Furthermore, there is growing evidence that social cognition mediates the relation between neurocognition and functional status in schizophrenia [22, 136] (also see chapter 2 of this volume). Hence, like basic neurocognition, social cognition is a determinant of functional outcome that appears to be a valuable target for intervention.

We would be remiss without acknowledging the advances in cognitive and affective neuroscience that have taken place over the past 2 decades that have led to the development of new behavioral methods for assessing neurocognitive function, social cognition and their underlying neural mechanisms [137–139]. The current review of measurement of neurocognition and social cognition reflects the best efforts of the field at this time. However, a priority for future research will be to expand the boundaries of assessment and entertain new models and methods. Findings from the neuroscience literature point towards promising new paradigms that may shed light on understanding the neurocognitive and social cognitive deficits associated with schizophrenia and their relationships with underlying brain mechanisms. These methods may ultimately lead to a pathway by which to assess new pharmacological treatments. First, there is the need for rigorous evaluation, but there is promise that measurement more proximal to the neural circuitry associated with selected neurocognitive and social cognitive deficits may eventually lead to fruitful treatments.

References

1 Kraepelin E: Dementia Praecox and Paraphrenia. Huntington, Krieger Publishing Co Inc, 1971.

2 Harvey P, Sharma T: Understanding and Treating Cognition in Schizophrenia: A Clinician's Handbook. London, Dunitz Ltd, 2002.

3 Nuechterlein KH, Barch DM, Gold JM, Goldberg TE, Green MF, Heaton RK: Identification of separable cognitive factors in schizophrenia. Schizophr Res 2004;72:29–39.

4 Gold J: Cognitive deficits as treatment targets in schizophrenia. Schizophr Res 2004;72:21–28.

5 Palmer B, Heaton, RK, Paulsen JS, Kuck J, Braff D, Harris MJ, Zisook S, Jeste DV: Is it possible to be schizophrenic yet neuropsychologically normal? Neuropsychology 1997;11:437–446.

6 Heinrichs RW, Zakzanis KK: Neurocognitive deficit in schizophrenia: a quantitative review of the evidence. Neuropsychology 1998;12:426–445.

7 Saykin AJ, Gur RC, Gur RE, Mozley PD, Mozley LH, Resnick SM, Kester DB, Stafiniak P: Neuropsychological function in schizophrenia: selective impairment in memory and learning. Arch Gen Psychiatry 1991;48:618–624.

8 Mohamed S, Paulsen JS, O'Leary DS, Arndt S, Andreasen NC: Generalized cognitive deficits in schizophrenia. Am J Psychiatry 1999;156:749–754.

9 Nieuwenstein MR, Aleman A, de Haan EHF: Relationship between symptom dimensions and neurocognitive functioning in schizophrenia: a meta-analysis of WCST and CPT studies. J Psychiatr Res 2001;35:119–125.

10 Heydebrand G, Weiser M, Rabinowitz J, Hoff AL, DeLisi LE, Csernansky JG: Correlates of cognitive deficits in first episode schizophrenia. Schizophr Res 2004;68:1–9.

11 Bilder RM, Goldman RS, Robinson D, Reiter G, Bell L, Bates JA, Pappadopulos E, Wilson DF, Alvir JM, Woerner MG, Geisler S, Kane JM, Lieberman JA: Neuropsychology of first-episode schizophrenia: initial characterization and clinical correlates. Am J Psychiatry 2000;157:549–559.

12 Addington J, Addington D, Maticka-Tyndale E: Cognitive functioning and positive and negative symptoms in schizophrenia. Schizophr Res 1991;5:123–134.

13 Addington J: Cognitive functioning and negative symptoms in schizophrenia; in Sharma T, Harvey P (eds): Cognition in Schizophrenia. Oxford, Oxford University Press, 2000, pp 193–209.

14 Nuechterlein KH, Asarnow RF, Subotnik KL, Fogelson DL, Ventura J, Torquato R, Dawson ME: Neurocognitive vulnerability factors for schizophrenia: convergence across genetic risk studies and longitudinal trait/state studies; in Lenzenweger MF, Dworkin RH (eds): Origins and Development of Schizophrenia: Advances in Experimental Psychopathology. Washington, American Psychological Association, 1998, pp 299–327.

15 Cornblatt B, Lenzenweger MF, Dworkin R, Erlenmeyer-Kimling L: Childhood attentional dysfunction predicts social deficits in unaffected adults at risk for schizophrenia. Br J Psychiatry 1992;161:59–64.

16 Bilder RM, Goldman RS, Volavka J, Czobor P, Hoptman M, Sheitman B, Lindenmayer J-P, Citrome L, McEvoy J, Kunz M, Chakos M, Cooper TB, Horowitz TL, Lieberman JA: Neurocognitive effects of clozapine, olanzapine, risperidone, and haloperidol in patients with chronic schizophrenia and schizoaffective disorder. Am J Psychiatry 2002;159:1018–1028.

17 Harvey PD, Keefe RSE: Studies of the cognitive change in patients with schizophrenia following novel antipsychotic treatment. Am J Psychiatry 2001;158:176–184.

18 Keefe RSE, Silva SG, Perkins DO, Lieberman JA: The effects of atypical antipsychotic drugs on neurocognitive impairment in schizophrenia: a review and meta-analysis. Schizophr Bull 1999;25:201–222.

19 Woodward ND, Purdon SE, Meltzer HY, Zald DH: A meta-analysis of neuropsychological change to clozapine, olanzapine, quetiapine, and risperidone in schizophrenia Int J Neuropsychopharmacol 2005;8:457–472.

20 Green MF, Marder SR, Glynn SM, McGurk SR, Wirshing WC, Wirshing DA, Liberman RP, Mintz J: The neurocognitive effects of low-dose haloperidol: a two-year comparison with risperidone. Biol Psychiatry 2002;51:972–978.

21 Green MF: What are the functional consequences of neurocognitive deficits in schizophrenia? Am J Psychiatry 1996;153:321–330.

22 Green MF, Kern RS, Braff DL, Mintz J: Neurocognitive deficits and functional outcome in schizophrenia: are we measuring the 'right stuff'? Schizophr Bull 2000;26:119–136.

23 Green MF, Kern RS, Heaton RK: Longitudinal studies of cognition and functional outcome in schizophrenia: implications for MATRICS. Schizophr Res 2004;72:41–51.

24 Nuechterlein KH, Green MF: MATRICS Consensus Cogntive Battery. Los Angeles, MATRICS Assessment Inc, 2006.

25 Reitan R, Wolfson D: The Halstead-Reitan Neuropsychological Test Battery: Theory and Clinical Interpretation, ed 2. Tuscon, Neuropsychology Press, 1993.

26 Army Individual Test Battery: Manual of Directions and Scoring. Washington, Adjutant General's Office, War Department, 1944.

27 Heaton RK: Wisconsin Card Sorting Test Manual. Odessa, Psychological Assessment Resources Inc, 1993.

28 Harvey P, Keefe R: Cognitive impairment in schizophrenia and the implications of atypical neuroleptic treatment. CNS Spectr 1997;2:41–55.

29 Keefe RSE: Brief Assessment of Cognition in Schizophrenia (BACS) Manual – A: Version 2.1. Durham, Duke University Medical Center, 1999.

30 Gold JM, Queern C, Iannone VN, Buchanan RW: Repeatable battery for the assessment of neuropsychological status as a screening test in schizophrenia. I. Sensitivity, reliability, and validity. Am J Psychiatry 1999;156:1944–1950.

31 Keefe R, Goldberg T, Harvey P, Gold J, Poe M, Coughenour L: The brief assessment of cognition in schizophrenia: reliability, sensitivity, and comparison with a standard neurocognitive battery. Schizophr Res 2004;68:283–297.

32 Kern RS, Green MF, Marshall BD, Wirshing WC, Wirshing D, McGurk S, Marder S, Mintz J: Risperidone vs. haloperidol on secondary memory: can newer antipsychotic medications aid learning? Schizophr Bull 1999;25:223–232.

33 Morris R, Evenden J, Sahakian B, Robbins T: Computer-aided assessment of dementia: comparative studies of neuropsychological deficits in Alzheimer-type dementia and Parkinson's disease; in Stahl S, Iversen S, Goodman E (eds): Cognitive Neurochemistry. Oxford, Oxford University Press, 1986, pp 21–36.

34 Levaux M, Potvin S, Sepehry A, Sablier J, Mendrek A, Stip E: Computerized assessment of cognition in schizophrenia: promises and pitfalls of CANTAB. Eur Psychiatry 2007;22:104–115.

35 Elwood R: Microcog: Assessment of cognitive functioning. Neuropsychol Rev 2001;11:89–100.

36 Baker E, Letz R, Fidler A, Shalat S, Plantamura D, Lyndon M: Computer-based neurobehavioral evaluation system for occupational and environmental epidemiology: methodology and validation studies. Neurobehav Toxicol Teratol 1985;7:369–377.

37 Silverstein SM, Berten S, Olson P, Paul R, Willams LM, Cooper N, Gordon E: Development and validation of a World-Wide-Web-based neurocognitive assessment battery: Webneuro. Behav Res Methods 2007;39:940–949.

38 Gur R, Ragland J, Moberg P, Turner T, Bilker W, Kohler C, Siegel S, Gur R: Computerized neurocognitive scanning. I. Methodology and validation in healthy people. Neuropsychopharmacology 2001;25:766–776.

39 Gur R, Ragland J, Moberg P, Bilker W, Kohler C, Siegel S, Gur R: Computerized neurocognitive scanning. II. The profile of schizophrenia. Neuropsychopharmacology 2001;25:777–788.

40 Williams LM, Whitford TJ, Flynn G, Wong W, Liddell BJ, Silverstein S, Galletly C, Harris AW, Gordon E: General and social cognition in first-episode schizophrenia: identification of separable factors and prediction of functional outcome using the Integneuro test battery. Schizophr Res 2008;99: 182–191.

41 Cysique L, Maruff P, Darby D, Brew B: The assessment of cognitive function in advanced HIV-1 infection and AIDS dementia complex using a new computerised cognitive test battery. Archi Clin Neuropsychol 2006;21:185–194.

42 Harvey P, Hassman H, Mao L, Gharabawi G, Mahmoud R, Engelhart L: Cognitive functioning and acute sedative effects of risperidone and quetiapine in patients with stable bipolar I disorder: a randomized, double-blind, crossover study. J Clin Psychiatry 2007;68:1186–1194.

43 Ritsner M, Blumenkrantz H, Dubinsky T, Dwolatzky T: The detection of neurocognitive decline in schizophrenia using the Mindstreams Computerized Cognitive Test Battery. Schizophr Res 2006;82:39–49.

44 O'Halloran J, Kemp A, Gooch K, Harvey P, Palmer B, Reist C, Schneider L: Psychometric comparison of computerized and standard administration of the neurocognitive assessment instruments selected by the CATIE and MATRICS consortia among patients with schizophrenia. Schizophr Res 2008;106:33–41.

45 Pantelis C, Barnes T, Nelson H, Tanner S, Weatherly L, Owen A, Robbins T: Frontal-striatal cognitive deficits in patients with chronic schizophrenia. Brain 1997;120:1823–1843.

46 Pietrzak R, Oliver J, Norman T, Piskulic C, Maruff P, Snyder P: A comparison of the Cogstate Schizophrenia Battery and the Measurement and Treatment Research to Improve Cognition in Schizophrenia (MATRICS) battery in assessing cognitive impairment in chronic schizophrenia. J Clin Exp Neuropsychol 2009;14:1–12.

47 American Psychological Association: Guidelines for Computer-Based Tests and Interpretation. Washington, American Psychological Association, 1986.

48 Kane R, Kay G: Computerized assessment in neuropsychology: a review of tests and test batteries. Neuropsychol Rev 1992;3:1–117.

49 Green MF, Nuechterlein KH, Gold JM, Barch DM, Cohen J, Essock S, Fenton WS, Frese F, Goldberg TE, Heaton RK, Keefe RSE, Kern RS, Kraemer H, Stover E, Weinberger DR, Zalcman S, Marder SR: Approaching a consensus cognitive battery for clinical trials in schizophrenia: the NIMH-MATRICS conference to select cognitive domains and test criteria. Biol Psychiatry 2004;56:301–307.

50 Marder SR, Fenton WS: Measurement and treatment research to improve cognition in schizophrenia: NIMH MATRICS initiative to support the development of agents for improving cognition in schizophrenia. Schizophr Res 2004;72:5–10.

51 Nuechterlein K, Green M, Kern RS, Baade L, Barch D, Cohen J, Essock S, Fenton W, Frese IF, Gold J, Goldberg T, Heaton R, Keefe R, Kraemer H, Mesholam-Gately R, Seidman L, Stover E, Weinberger D, Young A, Zalcman S, Marder S: The MATRICS Consensus Cognitive Battery. 1. Test selection, reliability, and validity. Am J Psychiatry 2008;165:203–213.

52 Holmen A, Juuhl-Langseth M, Thormodsen R, Melle I, Rund B: Neuropsychological profile in early-onset schizophrenia-spectrum disorders: measured with the MATRICS battery. Schizophr Bull, in press (epub available ahead of print).

53 Adolphs R: The neurobiology of social cognition. Curr Opin Neurobiol 2001;11:231–239.

54 Brothers L: The neural basis of primate social communication. Motiv Emot 1990;14:81–91.

55 Kunda Z: Social Cognition. Making Sense of People. Cambridge, MIT Press, 1999.

56 Fiske ST, Taylor SE: Social Cognition, ed 2. New York, McGraw-Hill Book Company, 1991.

57 Lieberman MD: Social cognitive neuroscience: a review of core processes. Annu Rev Psychol 2007;58:259–289.

58 Adolphs R: The social brain: neural basis of social knowledge. Annu Rev Psychol 2009;60:693–716.

59 Green MF, Penn DL, Bentall R, Carpenter WT, Gaebel W, Gur RC, Kring AM, Park S, Silverstein SM, Heinssen R: Social cognition in schizophrenia: an NIMH workshop on definitions, assessment, and research opportunities. Schizophr Bull 2008;34:1211–1220.

60 Mayer JD, Salovey P, Caruso DR, Sitarenios G: Emotional intelligence as a standard intelligence. Emotion 2001;1:232–242.

61 Salovey P, Sluyter DJ: Emotional Development and Emotional Intelligence. New York, Basic Books, 1997.

62 Kohler CG, Walker JB, Martin EA, Healey KM, Moberg PJ: Facial emotion perception in schizophrenia: a meta-analytic review. Schizophr Bull, in press (epub available ahead of print).

63 Kee KS, Horan WP, Mintz J, Green MF: Do the siblings of schizophrenia patients demonstrate affect perception deficits? Schizophr Res 2004;67:87–94.

64 Gur RE, Nimgaonkar VL, Almasy L, Calkins ME, Ragland JD, Pogue-Geile MF, Kanes S, Blangero J, Gur RC: Neurocognitive endophenotypes in a multiplex multigenerational family study of schizophrenia. Am J Psychiatry 2007;164:813–819.

65 Edwards J, Jackson HJ, Pattison PE: Emotional recognition via facial expression and affective prosody in schizophrenia: a methodological review. Clin Psychol Rev 2002;22:789–832.

66 Addington J, Penn DL, Woods SW, Addington D, Perkins DO: Facial affect recognition in individuals at clinical high risk for psychosis. Br J Psychiatry 2008;192:67–68.

67 Penn DL, Combs DR, Ritchie M, Francis J, Cassisi J, Morris S, Townsend M: Emotion recognition in schizophrenia: further investigation of generalized versus specific deficit models. J Abnorm Psychol 2000;109:512–516.

68 Mueser KT, Penn DL, Blanchard JJ, Bellack AS: Affect recognition in schizophrenia: a synthesis of findings across three studies. Psychiatry 1997;60:301–308.

69 Schneider F, Gur RC, Koch K, Backes V, Amunts K, Shah NJ, Bilker W, Gur RE, Habel U: Impairment in the specificity of emotion processing in schizophrenia. Am J Psychiatry 2006;163:442–447.

70 Kohler CG, Turner TH, Bilker WB, Brensinger CM, Siegel SJ, Kanes SJ, Gur RE, Gur RC: Facial emotion recognition in schizophrenia: intensity effects and error pattern. Am J Psychiatry 2003;160:1768–1774.

71 Johnston PJ, Enticott PG, Mayes AK, Hoy KE, Herring SE, Fitzgerald PB: Symptom correlates of static and dynamic facial affect processing in schizophrenia: evidence of double dissociation? Schizophr Bull, in press (epub available ahead of print).

72 McDonald S, Flanagan S, Rollins J: The Awareness of Social Inference Test. Suffolk, Thames Valley Test Company Ltd, 2002.

73 Couture SM, Penn DL, Roberts DL: The functional significance of social cognition in schizophrenia: a review. Schizophr Bull 2006;32(suppl 1):S44–S63.

74 Mayer JD, Salovey P, Caruso DR, Sitarenios G: Measuring emotional intelligence with the MSCEIT v2.0. Emotion 2003;3:97–105.

75 Eack SM, Greeno CG, Pogue-Geile MF, Newhill CE, Hogarty GE, Keshavan MS: Assessing social-cognitive deficits in schizophrenia with the Mayer-Salovey-Caruso emotional intelligence test. Schizophr Bull, in press (epub available ahead of print).

76 Kee KS, Horan WP, Salovey P, Kern RS, Sergi MJ, Fiske AP, Lee J, Subotnik KL, Nuechterlein K, Sugar CA, Green MF: Emotional intelligence in schizophrenia. Schizophr Res 2009;107:61–68.

77 Henry JD, Green MJ, de Lucia A, Restuccia C, McDonald S, O'Donnell M: Emotion dysregulation in schizophrenia: reduced amplification of emotional expression is associated with emotional blunting. Schizophr Res 2007;95:197–204.

78 Henry JD, Rendell PG, Green MJ, McDonald S, O'Donnell M: Emotion regulation in schizophrenia: affective, social, and clinical correlates of suppression and reappraisal. J Abnorm Psychol 2008;117: 473–478.

79 Horan WP, Blanchard JJ, Clark LA, Green MF: Affective traits in schizophrenia and schizotypy. Schizophr Bull 2008;34:856–874.

80 Corrigan PW, Green MF: Schizophrenic patients' sensitivity to social cues: the role of abstraction. Am J Psychiatry 1993;150:589–594.

81 Corrigan PW, Wallace CJ, Green MF: Deficits in social schemata in schizophrenia. Schizophr Res 1992;8:129–135.

82 Rosenthal R, Hall JA, DiMatteo MR, Rogers PL, Archer D: Sensitivity to Nonverbal Communication. The Pons Test. Baltimore, Johns Hopkins University Press, 1979.

83 Sergi MJ, Green MF: Social perception and early visual processing in schizophrenia. Schizophr Res 2002;59:233–241.

84 Corrigan PW, Davies-Farmer RM, Stolley MR: Social cue recognition in schizophrenia under variable levels of arousal. Cogn Ther Res 1990;14:353–361.

85 Addington J, Saeedi H, Addington D: Influence of social perception and social knowledge on cognitive and social functioning in early psychosis. Br J Psychiatry 2006;189:373–378.

86 Toomey R, Seidman LJ, Lyons MJ, Faraone SV, Tsuang MT: Poor perception of nonverbal social-emotional cues in relatives of schizophrenic patients. Schizophr Res 1999;40:121–130.

87 Monkul ES, Green MJ, Barrett JA, Robinson JL, Velligan DI, Glahn DC: A social cognitive approach to emotional intensity judgment deficits in schizophrenia. Schizophrenia Research 2007;94:245–252.

88 Green MJ, Waldron JH, Coltheart M: Emotional context processing is impaired in schizophrenia. Cogn Neuropsychiatry 2007;12:259–280.

89 Sasson N, Tsuchiya N, Hurley R, Couture SM, Penn DL, Adolphs R, Piven J: Orienting to social stimuli differentiates social cognitive impairment in autism and schizophrenia. Neuropsychologia 2007;45:2580–2588.

90 Bigelow NO, Paradiso S, Adolphs R, Moser DJ, Arndt S, Heberlein A, Nopoulos P, Andreasen NC: Perception of socially relevant information in schizophrenia. Schizophrenia Research 2006;83:257–267.

91 Corrigan PW, Green MF: Schizophrenic patients' sensitivity to social cues: the role of abstraction. Am J Psychiatry 1993;150:589–594.

92 Subotnik KL, Nuechterlein KH, Green MF, Horan WP, Nienow TM, Ventura J, Nguyen AT: Neurocognitive and social cognitive correlates of formal thought disorder in schizophrenia patients. Schizophr Res 2006;85:84–95.

93 Corrigan PW, Green MF: The situational feature recognition test: a measure of schema comprehension for schizophrenia. Int J Meth Psychiatr Res 1993;3:29–35.

94 Corrigan PW, Addis I: The effects of cognitive complexity on a social sequencing task in schizophrenia. Schizophr Res 1995;16:137–144.

95 Penn DL, Ritchie M, Francis J, Combs D, Martin J: Social perception in schizophrenia: the role of context. Psychiatry Res 2002;109:149–159.

96 Bellack AS, Sayers M, Mueser K, Bennett M: Evaluation of social problem solving in schizophrenia. J Abnor Psychol 1994;103:371–378.

97 Kinderman P, Bentall RP: A new measure of causal locus: the internal, personal, and situational attributions questionnaire. Pers Individ Dif 1996;20:261–264.

98 Lee DA, Randall F, Beattie G, Bentall RP: Delusional discourse: an investigation comparing the spontaneous causal attributions of paranoid and non-paranoid individuals. Psychol Psychother 2004;77:525–540.

99 Bentall RP, Corcoran R, Howard R, Blackwood N, Kinderman P: Persecutory delusions: a review and theoretical integration. Clin Psychol Rev 2001;21: 1143–1192.

100 Garety PA, Freeman D: Cognitive approaches to delusions: a critical review of theories and evidence. Br J Clin Psychol 1999;38:113–154.

101 Peterson C, Semmel A, von Baeyer C, Abramson L, Metalsky GI, Seligman MEP: The attributional style questionnaire. Cogn Ther Res 1982;3:287–300.

102 Bentall RP, Corcoran R, Howard R, Blackwood N, Kinderman P: Persecutory delusions: a review and theoretical integration. Clin Psychol Rev 2001;21: 1143–1192.

103 Combs DR, Penn DL, Wicher M, Waldheter E: The Ambiguous Intentions Hostility Questionnaire (AIHQ): a new measure for evaluating hostile social-cognitive biases in paranoia. Cogn Neuropsychiatry 2007;12:128–143.

104 Stratton P, Munton AG, Hanks H, Heard DH, Davidson C: Leeds Attributional Coding System. Leeds, Leeds Family Research Centre, 1988.

105 Aakre JM, Seghers JP, St-Hilaire A, Docherty NM: Attributional style in delusional patients: a comparison of remitted paranoid, remitted nonparanoid, and current paranoid patients with nonpsychiatric controls. Schizophr Bull 2009;35:994–1002.

106 Baron-Cohen S, Wheelwright S, Hill J, Raste Y, Plumb I: The 'Reading the Mind in the Eyes' Test revised version: a study with normal adults, and adults with Asperger syndrome or high-functioning autism. J Child Psychol Psychiatry Allied Disc 2001; 42:241–251.

107 Frith CD: The Cognitive Neuropsychology of Schizophrenia. Hove, Lawrence Erlbaum Associates, Publishers, 1992.

108 Frith CD, Corcoran R: Exploring 'theory of mind' in people with schizophrenia. Psychol Med 1996;26: 521–530.

109 Corcoran R, Mercer G, Frith CD: Schizophrenia, symptomatology and social inference: investigating 'theory of mind' in people with schizophrenia. Schizophr Res 1995;17:5–13.

110 Baron-Cohen S, Wheelwright S, Hill J, Raste Y, Plumb I: The 'Reading the Mind in the Eyes' Test revised version: a study with normal adults, and adults with Asperger syndrome or high-functioning autism. J Child Psychol Psychiatry Allied Disc 2001; 42:241–251.

111 Langdon R, Michie PT, Ward PB, McConaghy N, Catts S, Coltheart M: Defective self and/or other mentalising in schizophrenia: a cognitive neuropsychological approach. Cogn Neuropsychiatry 1997;2: 167–193.

112 Happe F: An advanced test of theory of mind: Understanding of story characters' thoughts and feelings by able autistic, mentally handicapped and normal children and adults. J Autism Dev Disord 1994;24:129–154.

113 Brune M: Social cognition and behaviour in schizophrenia; in Brune M, Ribbert H, Schiefenhovel W (eds): The Social Brain-Evolution of Psychology. Chichester, Wiley & Sons, 2003, pp 277–313.

114 Corcoran R: Theory of mind and schizophrenia; in Corrigan PW, Penn DL (eds): Social Cognition and Schizophrenia. Washington, American Psychological Association, 2001, pp 149–174.

115 Brüne M: 'Theory of mind' in schizophrenia: a review of the literature Schizophr Bull 2005;31:21–42.

116 Bora E, Yucel M, Panteli C: Theory of mind impairment in schizophrenia: Meta-analysis. Schizophr Res 2009;109:1–9.

117 Sprong M, Schothorst P, Vos E, Hox J, Van Engeland H: Theory of mind in schizophrenia: meta-analysis. Br J Psychiatry 2007;191:5–13.

118 Chung YS, Kang DH, Shin NY, Yoo SY, Kwon JS: Deficit of theory of mind in individuals at ultrahigh-risk for schizophrenia. Schizophr Res 2008;99: 111–118.

119 Marjoram D, Miller P, McIntosh AM, Cunningham Owens DG, Johnstone EC, Lawrie S: A neuropsychological investigation into 'theory of mind' and enhanced risk of schizophrenia. Psychiatry Res 2006; 144:29–37.

120 Pinkham AE, Penn DL: Neurocognitive and social cognitive predictors of interpersonal skill in schizophrenia. Psychiatry Res 2006;143:167–178.

121 Kern RS, Green MF, Fiske AP, Kee KS, Lee J, Sergi MJ, Horan WP, Subotnik KL, Sugar CA, Nuechterlein KH: Theory of mind deficits for processing counterfactual information in persons with chronic schizophrenia. Psychol Med 2009;39:645–654.

122 Horan WP, Nuechterlein KH, Wynn JK, Lee J, Castelli F, Green MF: Disturbances in the spontaneous attribution of social meaning in schizophrenia. Psychol Med 2009;39:635–643.

123 Hegarty JD, Baldessarini RJ, Tohen M, Waternaux C, Oepen G: One hundred years of schizophrenia: a meta-analysis of the outcome literature. Am J Psychiatry 1994;151:1409–1416.

124 Baron R, Salzer M: Accounting for unemployment among people with mental illness. Behav Sci Law 2002;20:585–599.

125 Kooyman I, Dean K, Harvey S, Walsh E: Outcomes of public concern in schizophrenia. Br J Psychiatry Suppl 2007;50:s29–s36.

126 Yager J, Ehmann T: Untangling social function and social cognition: a review of concepts and measurement. Psychiatry 2006;69:47–68.

127 Green MF, Olivier B, Crawley JN, Penn DL, Silverstein S: Social cognition in schizophrenia: recommendations from the MATRICS new approaches conference. Schizophr Bull 2005;31:882–887.

128 Penn DL, Corrigan PW, Bentall RP, Racenstein JM, Newman L: Social cognition in schizophrenia. Psychol Bull 1997;121:114–132.

129 Penn DL, Spaulding WD, Reed D, Sullivan M: The relationship of social cognition to ward behavior in chronic schizophrenia. Schizophr Res 1996;20:327–335.

130 Sergi MJ, Rassovsky Y, Widmark C, Reist C, Erhart S, Braff DL, Marder SR, Green MF: Social cognition in schizophrenia: relationships with neurocognition and negative symptoms. Schizophr Res 2007;90:316–324.

131 Pinkham AE, Penn DL, Perkins DO, Lieberman J: Implications for the neural basis of social cognition for the study of schizophrenia. Am J Psychiatry 2003;160:815–824.

132 Brunet-Gouet E, Decety J: Social brain dysfunctions in schizophrenia: a review of neuroimaging studies. Psychiatry Res 2006;148:75–92.

133 Jones W, Bellugih U, Lai Z, Chiles M, Reilly J, Lincoln A, Adolphs R: II: Hypersociability in Williams syndrome. J Cogn Neurosci 2000;12:30–46.

134 Anderson SW, Bechara A, Damasio H, Tranel D, Damasio AR: Impairment of social and moral behavior related to early damage in human prefrontal cortex. Nat Neurosci 1999;2:1032–1037.

135 Kanwisher N: Domain specificity in face perception. Nat Neurosci 2000;3:759–763.

136 Green MF, Nuechterlein KH: Should schizophrenia be treated as a neurocognitive disorder? Schizophr Bull 1999;25:309–319.

137 Barch DM, Carter CS, Arnsten A, Buchanan RW, Cohen JD, Geyer M, Green MF, Krystal JH, Nuechterlein K, Robbins T, Silverstein S, Smith EE, Strauss M, Wykes T, Heinssen R: Selecting paradigms from cognitive neuroscience for translation into use in clinical trials: proceedings of the third CNTRICS meeting. Schizophr Bull 2009;35:109–114.

138 Ochsner KN: The social-emotional processing stream: five core constructs and their translational potential for schizophrenia and beyond. Biol Psychiatry 2008;64:48–61.

139 Carter CS, Barch DM, Gur R, Pinkham A, Ochsner K: CNTRICS final task selection: social cognitive and affective neuroscience-based measures. Schizophr Bull 2009;35:153–162.

140 Cornblatt B, Risch N, Faris G, Friedman D, Erlenmeyer-Kimling L: The continuous performance test-identical pairs (CPT-IP). I. New findings about sustained attention in normal families. Psychiatry Res 1988;26:223–238.

141 Cornblatt BA, Lenzenweger MF, Erlenmeyer-Kimling L: The continuous performance test, identical pairs version. II. Contrasting attentional profiles in schizophrenic and depressed patients. Psychiatr Res 1989;29:65.

142 Spreen O, Strauss E: A Compendium of Neuropsychological Tests. New York, Oxford University Press, 1991.

143 Gold JM, Carpenter C, Randolph C, Goldberg TE, Weinberger DR: Auditory working memory and Wisconsin card sorting test performance in schizophrenia. Arch Gen Psychiatry 1997;54:159–165.

144 Wechsler D: Wechsler Memory Scale, ed 3. San Antonio, Psychological Corporation, 1997.

145 Brandt J, Benedict RHB: The Hopkins Verbal Learning Test – Revised: Professional Manual. Odessa, Psychological Assessment Resources Inc, 2001.

146 Benedict RHB: Brief Visuospatial Memory Test – Revised: Professional Manual. Odessa, Psychological Assessment Resources Inc, 1997.

147 White T, Stern RA: Neuropsychological Assessment Battery: Psychometric and Technical Manual. Lutz, Psychological Assessment Resources Inc, 2003.

148 Kerr SL, Neale JM: Emotion perception in schizophrenia: specific deficit or further evidence of generalized poor performance? J Abnorm Psychol 1993;102:312–318.

Robert S. Kern, PhD
VA Greater Los Angeles Healthcare System (MIRECC 210 A)
Building 210, Room 116, 11301 Wilshire Blvd.
Los Angeles, CA 90073 (USA)
Tel. +1 310 478 3711, ext.49229, Fax +1 310 268 4056, E-Mail rkern@ucla.edu

Roder V, Medalia A (eds): Neurocognition and Social Cognition in Schizophrenia Patients. Basic Concepts and Treatment. Key Issues Ment Health. Basel, Karger, 2010, vol 177, pp 23–36

2
_____

The Relevance of Neurocognition and Social Cognition for Outcome and Recovery in Schizophrenia

John S. Brekke · Eri Nakagami

School of Social Work, University of Southern California, Los Angeles, Calif., USA

_____

Abstract

Over a decade of research has shown that neurocognition and social cognition are highly relevant to functional outcome in schizophrenia. These 2 factors can function as predictors, mediators or moderators of functioning under various conditions. One purpose of this chapter will be to summarize this body of literature. The notion of recovery in schizophrenia does not yet have a consensus or gold standard definition, and there appear to be at least 2 domains to recovery, the functional and the subjective. These 2 domains reflect somewhat distinct ideologies and approaches to outcome in schizophrenia. In fact, it appears that there is a stakeholder effect in the definitions of recovery, with clinicians and researchers focusing more on the functional aspects of recovery, and advocates and consumers more on the subjective ones. A second task of this chapter will be to address how neurocognition and social cognition are relevant to the notion of recovery in schizophrenia. Finally, we will offer speculation about conceptual approaches to research on recovery in schizophrenia.

Over a decade of research has shown that neurocognition and social cognition are highly relevant to functional outcome in schizophrenia. These 2 factors can function as predictors, mediators or moderators of functioning under various conditions. One purpose of this chapter will be to summarize this body of literature. However, functional outcome and recovery are not synonymous in at least 2 ways. First, there is some growing consensus on what dimensions of functional outcome are most relevant in schizophrenia. This is not the case with regard to the concept of recovery; in fact, it appears that there is a stakeholder effect in the definitions of recovery, with clinicians and researchers focusing more on the functional aspects of recovery, and advocates and consumers more on the subjective factors. A second task of this chapter will be to address how neurocognition and social cognition are relevant to the notion of recovery in schizophrenia.

Recovery and Outcome in Schizophrenia

Ever since the US President's New Freedom Commission Report [1] strongly urged the adoption of the notion of recovery as possible for all and as the guiding vision for mental health services, much effort has been placed in transforming services to achieve recovery outcomes. Although the notion of recovery has begun guiding policies and practices in many mental health systems in the USA, consensus has not been as strong regarding how to define and measure recovery. The definitions of recovery vary greatly between individuals and among groups including consumers, family members, clinicians and researchers which have evolved from distinct perspectives, historical contexts and goals [2]. The definitions of recovery differ between objective and subjective referents [3–5] as well as between recovery as an outcome and recovery as a process [6–8].

The scientific definitions of recovery began with the view that mental illness has a mainly biological etiology and placed the goal of recovery to be the complete absence of the illness, a cure and a return to normal life functioning. Over time, it has been recognized that recovery might not need to imply a cure and that enduring symptoms may fluctuate within a certain range [3]. Furthermore, the notion of functional heterogeneity with regard to recovery is applicable, since the relationship between symptoms and functioning in residual or chronic phases of the disorder is modest at best [9]. For example, one individual may experience relatively severe symptoms but function moderately well in employment, while others may have mild symptoms and not function well in their daily activities.

It has also been acknowledged that recovery involves subjective experiences and defining what is 'normal' functioning entails several value judgments, since unlike cognitive performance, there is no gold standard for functional outcomes [3]. Nonetheless, scientific definitions have continued to view recovery as an outcome and focus on clinical symptoms and functioning such as '...the performance of daily activities that are required for self-maintenance (earning an income and maintain a residence), as well as social activities' [3], which include a protracted period (e.g. at least 6 months) of minimal symptoms (i.e. positive and negative symptoms), normal neuropsychiatric functioning and the ability for people to function independently in the real world [10].

Contrary to the more scientific approach, consumer definitions of recovery do not view recovery as an outcome but rather as a holistic nonlinear process of '…positive adaptation to illness and disability...' [11] moving beyond disability and pursuing a deeply personal and meaningful life that involves hope, empowerment, motivation, personal responsibility and independent goals. Consumer definitions of recovery also encompass human rights, combating stigma, community integration, discrimination, as well as promoting recovery-oriented practices, services and policies [11, 12]. As evidence of this, Brekke et al. [13] describe a stakeholder process for defining the outcomes from rehabilitation services in which consumers were sensitive to the functional aspects of recovery and outcome but were far more attached to the subjective aspects such as motivation, self-esteem, internalized stigma, hope and autonomy. In fact, they named these subjective aspects the 'core strengths' and argued that improvement in the core strengths was far more important to them than changes in the common functional outcomes of work and independent living.

While the scientific definition would describe an individual as recovering 'from' mental illness, which suggests an alleviation of the illness, the consumer definition would consider an individual as 'being in recovery', which implies progressing with life despite enduring symptoms [7]. Despite the differing definitions, there is consensus that there are multiple domains of recovery, individuals with schizophrenia are extremely heterogeneous in each aspects of recovery, and the realms are relatively independent from one another [4, 14].

Nonetheless, the attempt to separate outcome from process has led to 2 distinct research foci where the scientific view has attended mainly to the relationship between cognition and functional recovery, while the consumer view has emphasized the subjective experiences that play a part towards achieving a meaningful life. Some investigators have examined the relationships between functional recovery and subjective experiences [14], but there is a dearth of information on the empirical relationship between cognition, functional recovery, and the 'process' elements encompassed in consumer definitions of recovery such as hope, motivation, empowerment and independent goals.

While the scientific view has clearly dominated the research literature on outcome and recovery, Liberman and Kopelowicz [8] note that process and outcome are always in dynamic interaction with one another. Discerning how the subjective and process variables of recovery relate to cognition and functional outcomes would shed light on an area that is not well understood and would add significantly to the knowledge base and clinical interventions for individuals with schizophrenia.

Before turning to functional recovery, we would like to briefly address symptomatic aspects of recovery. The relationship of neurocognition to symptoms in schizophrenia is complex. There are cognitive models of schizophrenia that attempt to construct the core cognitive deficit or dysfunction that leads to the disorder, but they are challenged by symptom heterogeneity across individuals and time [15]. While neurocognition is related to negative symptoms [16], it has not been associated with symptomatic exacerbations or remission. In addition, compared with positive and negative symptoms, neurocognition appears to be a stronger predictor of functional outcomes [9, 17, 18]. Therefore, we are not including a discussion of neurocognition and symptomatic aspects of recovery. Given the high rates of medication noncompliance in schizophrenia, one productive avenue is to examine the neurocognitive correlates of medication compliance or of responsiveness to medication compliance interventions.

Functional Dimensions

Functional deficits in schizophrenia are a major cause of disability, accounting for a substantial portion of the indirect costs of the illness [19]. In the past few years, assessments of functional disability have attempted to delineate 3 dimensions of functioning in schizophrenia; functional capacity, functional performance and functional outcomes [20, 21]. Functional capacity refers to an individual's ability or competence in performing tasks of daily living (e.g. holding a conversation, preparing a meal, performing job-related tasks, taking public transportation), which are most often assessed in controlled settings such as testing labs or clinics [12, 22, 23]. Functional capacity tends to reflect the microskills of daily living tasks. While functional capacity is highly variable, it appears to be stable over time [4].

Functional performance refers to the individual's ability to perform or engage in the abovementioned behaviors in the real world, in their natural living environments. Lieberman et al. [4] note that functional performance has a changeable course with a considerable return of psychosocial functioning after initial episodes, an escalating deterioration after subsequent episodes and the possibility for a certain degree of functional improvement afterward. Functional outcomes are the result of both capacity and performance and are typically measured as a level of achievement in work, independent living and social domains that are occurring in the individual's natural living environments [24]. These are the more macrooutcomes such as the amount and type of work and money earned, the independence of living situations, or the breadth and type of social networks.

Evaluating the critical difference between what an individual is able to do and what they actually do in the real world is also referred to as the 'competence/performance distinction' [25]. The 3 dimensions of functioning emerged as it became clear that successfully demonstrating functional capacity does not necessarily mean that the individual will be able to perform the tasks in their own community settings. Individual characteristics such as motivation, confidence, risk-taking, self-evaluative abilities and environmental factors (e.g. social support, employment and housing opportunities) may at times have more influence on real-world performance than functional capacity alone. Studies have observed that although neuropsychological performance is highly associated with functional outcome [9, 18, 26, 27], the relationship between neuropsychological and functional performance has been found to be mediated by functional capacity [17]. Although these capacity measures present logistical advantages over other less direct methods of examining functional outcome, they do not always provide helpful information about community behavior [25].

While the empirical relationships between functional capacity, functional performance and other outcome constructs have not been widely studied, functional capacity appears to be influenced more by cognitive functioning, whereas functional performance and outcome are more determined by environmental factors [17, 18]. Thus, cognitive determinants can be modified or moderated by environmental determinants.

Cognitive Determinants of Functional Dimensions

Extensive research over the past 2 decades has demonstrated that individuals with schizophrenia have a variety of neurocognitive impairments including attention, episodic and working memory, language and problem-solving, which contribute considerably to the functional difficulties for individuals with schizophrenia [9, 18, 26–28]. These deficits are exhibited at the onset of the illness, are stable over time [29] and are modestly influenced by psychiatric medications [30]. Cognitive impairments have been found to predict self-care, social functioning, community-living skills and employment [31] cross-sectionally as well as longitudinally [32–34]. These deficits are better than positive symptoms for predicting functional outcomes [9, 18]. Further, several studies have found that impairments in different domains of cognition are associated with distinct functional outcomes: attention and vigilance with social functioning; memory and verbal learning with social, occupational and independent living; executive functioning with independent living; processing speed with employment [18, 35].

Two other areas in the study of neurocognition and functional outcome have recently emerged: neurocognitive change and cognitive remediation. Brekke et al. [13] studied neurocognitive and functional change during 1 year of community-based psychosocial rehabilitation for individuals with schizophrenia. They found a strong relationship between composite neurocognitive improvement and global functional improvement and further that there was an interaction between neurocognitive progress, service intensity and the rate of functional improvement such that service intensity was strongly related to functional development for neurocognitive improvers but not for neurocognitive nonimprovers. This suggests that neurocognitive improvement might be a foundation for functional change and treatment responsiveness in schizophrenia.

Cognitive remediation is based on the notion that improving cognition will enhance the functional outcomes. Given the importance of neurocognition to functioning and rehabilitative change, there has been a focus on interventions to improve neurocognition in schizophrenia. Two meta-analytic reviews of cognitive remediation interventions [35, 36] conclude that global neurocognition, and also many specific domains of neurocognition such as verbal working memory, can be improved by cognitive remediation. Based on the assumption that neurocognitive change could be a foundation for functional change, there have also been attempts to integrate cognitive remediation and psychosocial rehabilitation interventions [37–41]. In this regard, there is evidence from meta-analyses that adding cognitive remediation to existing psychosocial rehabilitation interventions produces greater cognitive and functional improvement than psychosocial intervention alone [36].

Despite the significant relationship between neurocognition and functional outcomes, the correlation between the 2 constructs is generally modest with composite measures of neurocognition accounting for roughly 20–60% of the variance in functioning outcome [9, 18]. This highly variable relationship has prompted investigators to search for other factors such as mediators and moderators that influence and clarify the relationship between neurocognition and functioning outcome.

Social Cognition and Functional Outcomes

Social cognition has been examined as both a predictor of functional outcomes, and as a promising mediator of neurocognition and functional outcome [32, 33, 42, 43]. Social cognition is defined as the mental operations that underlie social interactions such as perception, interpretation and generation of responses to the intentions, dispositions and behaviors of others [44–46]. Social cognitive processes are the way we draw inferences about other people's beliefs and intentions as well as how we consider the mental representations and social situations to make these inferences.

Social cognition encompasses various abilities, but the ones most frequently studied in persons with schizophrenia are perception of emotion, social perception, social knowledge, theory of mind and attributional style [46, 47]. Perception of emotion (also known as emotion perception and affect recognition) is the ability to infer emotional information (i.e. what a person is feeling) from facial expressions, vocal inflections or the combination of both. Social perception refers to a person's ability to ascertain social cues from behaviors provided in social contextual situations such as emotion cues. Social perception is closely linked to social knowledge, which is the person's comprehension of social rules and conventions that guide social interactions. The theory of mind (also known as mental state attribution) involves the ability to infer intentions, dispositions and beliefs of others. Attributional styles are causal statements that involve the word 'because' and reflect how individuals typically infer the causes of particular positive and negative events [47].

Studies have found an association between neurocognition and social cognition as well as a relationship between social cognition and functional outcome [46, 47]. The mediating role of social cognition and its indirect relationship with neurocognition and functioning outcome has been supported [32, 42, 43]. Different aspects of neurocognition such as early visual processing, verbal recognition memory, visual vigilance, executive functioning and sensorimotor gating have been found to associate with perception of emotion and social perception.

The neural foundations of neurocognitive and social cognitive abilities suggest semiindependent structures for processing nonsocial and social stimuli [48]. Thus, social cognition may contribute to functioning outcome in a manner that is not redundant with neurocognition [46]. Existing studies have found that the greatest social cognitive impairment for individuals with schizophrenia appears to be in the perception of emotion [49, 50]. Many persons with schizophrenia also present restricted visual scanning and spend less time examining salient facial features during perception of emotion tasks [51–53].

Other investigations have demonstrated that there is a consistent relationship between social perception and various aspects of functional outcome, especially social problem-solving, social behavior in the treatment milieu and community functioning [53, 54]. The relationship between social perception and social skill has been inconsistent but shows potential [46]. Perception of emotion seems to have a rather consistent relationship with community functioning [33], social behavior [53, 54] and vocational functioning [55]. Perception of emotion may also mediate the link between neurocognition and functional outcome [32]. There has been less research on functional outcome and theory of mind [56] or attributional style [57], but initial studies are promising.

Environmental Moderators of the Functional Dimensions

There are a host of factors that could intervene as mediators or moderators between neurocognition and functional outcome. It has been hypothesized that environmental characteristics could be moderating the relationship between neurocognition and functional outcomes [58]. Brekke [58] has suggested that 3 environmental determinants are potentially critical for functional performance to occur and for the functional outcome to improve and endure: opportunity, support and enhancements. Opportunities such as available options for housing, employment and social engagement must be in place. It is obvious that someone who has the functional capacity for work but who cannot find employment will have poor occupational outcomes. The same is true with regard to social functioning and housing. Second, the support of family, friends, peers and/or staff who encourage adaptive behaviors and behavioral change must also be available. These supports could be particularly significant for individuals who are struggling with long-standing psychiatric challenges and cycles of relapse and hospitalization. Finally, enhancements, such as available treatments or services that aim toward improving the functional outcome of persons with schizophrenia, are a significant environmental factor as well.

Figure 1 suggests that the cognitive determinants will have the most direct impact on indicators of functional capacity because environmental factors can be controlled and minimized in laboratory settings. Functional performance and outcome are more environmentally determined. Therefore, the influence of the cognitive determinants is modified or moderated by environmental factors [18, 25, 58]. While studies are needed to carefully test these notions, there is evidence that neurocognition is a stronger predictor of functional capacity than functional outcome [17, 18].

Neurocognition, Social Cognition and Recovery

As can be seen, a wealth of research has been conducted on neurocognition, social cognition and the scientific definition of recovery – namely the functional outcome

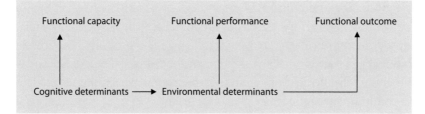

Fig. 1. The relationship between cognitive and environmental determinants of the functional dimensions.

domains of work, independent living and social relationships – for persons with schizophrenia. However, as noted before, the consumer definitions of recovery encompass the subjective and process-oriented factors such as hope, empowerment, motivation, quality of life, satisfaction with life, self-esteem, self-efficacy, personal responsibility and independent goals [11, 12]. Very little is known about how these subjective experience variables are associated with neurocognition, social cognition and the typical functional outcomes.

Brekke et al. [59] found that neurocognition moderated the relationship between functional outcome and the subjective indicators of self-esteem and satisfaction with life. Specifically, higher cognition was associated with a weak nonsignificant relationship between functional outcome and subjective satisfaction with self and life, while lower cognition was related to a strong and positive link between functional outcome level and subjective satisfaction. This suggests that when more subjective aspects of recovery are studied, neurocognition might have a less direct impact and serve more as an intervening or moderating factor.

Motivation has received considerable attention [60, 61] since the significance of understanding the motivational processes in schizophrenia was emphasized at the New Approaches to Cognition Conference [62]. Motivation difficulties, including amotivation, avolition and anhedonia, are components of negative symptoms of schizophrenia that have been found to mediate the relationship between symptoms and various functioning outcomes for persons with schizophrenia [63]. They are also one of the most frequent barriers to employment for people with psychiatric disabilities [64].

Motivation problems have generally been examined from a neurobiological perspective suggesting that motivation impairments are secondary to organic deterioration or that they result from neural deficits in brain centers that mediate phenomenal pleasure and behavioral reward [60]. However, these studies have not been consistent as some have demonstrated that external incentives enhance extrinsic motivation and increase cognitive performance even on characteristic markers of schizophrenia such as vigilance, span of apprehension and facial affect perception [65–67], while others have not found improvements in cognitive task performance for persons with schizophrenia [60].

Investigations into the cognitive mechanisms underlying extrinsic motivation, reward-based and reinforcement-learning tasks have elucidated an area that has been a perplexing one. Much more remains to be examined in this field, but recently the importance of understanding the neural mechanisms that underpin other aspects of motivation such as intrinsic motivation has been emphasized [60]. Towards that end, studies have found that intrinsic motivation mediates the relationship between cognition and functional outcome [60, 68, 69].

Research on motivation and outcome tested 2 models of the relationship between anhedonia, social perception and functional outcome and found that although anhedonia and social perception were not significantly correlated with each other, they were significantly associated with different aspects of functional outcome, leading Horan et al. [11] to conclude that motivational and social cognitive variables may be particularly important in elucidating the unexplained variance and predicting different aspects of functional outcome including work, social functioning and independent living. Alternatively, Sharma and Antova [70] assert that motivation difficulties may lead individuals to perform poorly on cognitive tasks in the laboratory and to fail to engage in or perform life functions necessary to live and work independently.

Using a Motivational Trait Questionnaire [71], Barch [72] found that individuals with schizophrenia did not differ from controls on personal mastery and competitive excellence but reported significantly higher motivation related to anxiety. Their results were not consistent with the theory that motivational deficits in schizophrenia suggest impairments in intrinsic motivation but did reflect that the normal relationship between self-reports of intrinsic motivation and cognitive function is disrupted in schizophrenia. More studies to ascertain the neural underpinnings that are associated with the various aspects of motivation along with the processes that lead to therapeutic change may help sort through the aspects that are particularly important in enhancing motivation and improving the treatment outcomes. These investigations may also identify the conditions on which the effectiveness of a given treatment may be contingent.

Working alliance is a factor that is broadly defined by Horvath [73] as the quality and strength of the collaborative relationship between client and therapist. This is mentioned as an important aspect of recovery by consumers [12]. Studies have found conflicting results between neurocognition and working alliance; poorer performance on verbal memory was significantly related to consumer appraisal of stronger alliance, while higher performance on spatial reasoning was significantly linked to provider evaluation of stronger alliance [74]. Neurocognitive impairment may lead to difficulties in interpersonal relationships [75] and thereby impair the formation of a therapeutic alliance.

Clearly, more research is needed on the relationship between neurocognition, social cognition and the subjective aspects of recovery in schizophrenia. Understanding how other process variables relate to cognition and functional outcomes has implications for the theoretical exlanation of the relationship between cognition, social cognition and psychosocial functioning in schizophrenia.

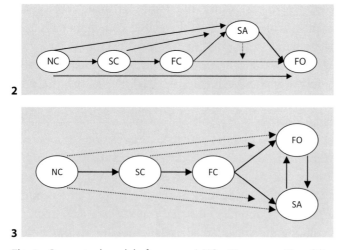

2

3

Fig. 2. Conceptual model of recovery I. NC = Neurocognition; SC = social cognition; FC = functional capacity; SA = subjective aspects; FO = functional outcome. Dotted lines reflect mediation or moderation.

Fig. 3. Conceptual model of recovery II. NC = Neurocognition; SC = social cognition; FC = functional capacity; SA = subjective aspects; FO = functional outcome. Dotted lines reflect effects that might occur in some models.

Conceptual Approaches to Research on Recovery in Schizophrenia

One approach to studying the neurocognitive and social cognitive mechanisms related to functional outcome and recovery is to eliminate the subjective aspects of these constructs from scientific consideration [24]. However, if we are to accept that these subjective aspects are central to recovery as the consumer perspective holds [2], then we need a program of research that integrates them into scientific consideration. Toward that end we offer 2 possible conceptual approaches to studying mechanisms of recovery in schizophrenia that include neurocognition, social cognition and both functional outcomes and subjective aspects of recovery.

The first model posits that subjective aspects of recovery such as empowerment, hope, internalized stigma, autonomy and self-esteem are intervening variables (either mediators or moderators) between neurocognition, social cognition, functional capacity and functional outcomes (see fig. 2). While this model proposes that neurocognition, social cognition and functional capacity are causally linked in the manner shown and they can have direct and indirect impact on both subjective aspects and functional outcome in recovery, it also suggests that the subjective aspects could either mediate or moderate in this causal chain. For example, hope might be a critical mediator of these relationships such that changes in functional outcome can be explained best by the impact of neurocognition, social cognition and functional capacity on hope. Alternately, the levels of hope might moderate these relationships such that improvements in functional outcome might be contingent on the presence of a certain level of hope. Any of the subjective variables, or perhaps a subjective construct consisting of a number of subjective variables, could be used in the same way in this conceptual model.

Another approach is offered in figure 3, which posits a model wherein neurocognition, social cognition and functional capacity all have direct and perhaps indirect effects on both the functional outcomes and the subjective aspects of recovery. Importantly, in this model the 2 aspects of recovery are seen as reciprocally influencing each other, such that the subjective aspects affect the functional outcomes and vice versa. This model also implies that perhaps there is a construct of recovery that includes both functional and subjective domains.

As a further speculation, these subjective aspects might be divided into subjective outcomes and subjective mechanisms. The subjective outcomes, such as satisfaction with life, self-concept and community integration can be seen as subjective endpoints for the assessment of treatment and recovery outcomes. Other variables might be called the subjective mechanisms, such as hope, internalized stigma, autonomy and self-directed goals. For example, rather than seeing hope as a subjective outcome, it might best be considered as a mediator or moderator of other outcomes, including the subjective ones such as satisfaction with life. Dividing the subjective factors in this fashion will clearly delineate which are aspects of recovery outcomes and which are mechanisms that will influence recovery outcomes.

These speculations are offered in the interest of beginning the discussion on how the concept of recovery can become a scientific construct that fully represents the multiple stakeholders in the mental health community including consumers, advocates, clinicians, administrators and policy makers. This will also facilitate developing biosocial models of recovery which include neurocognition, social cognition as well as environmental determinants in ways that will further the basic understanding of the course of the disorder, and contribute to understanding the effects of psychopharmacologic treatments and psychosocial interventions.

References

1 New Freedom Commission on Mental Health: Achieving the Promise: Transforming Mental Health Care in America. Final Report. DHHS pub No SMA-03-3832. Rockville Department of Health and Human Services, 2007. www.mentalhealthcommission.gov/reports/final report/fullreport-02.htm (retrieved January 4, 2007).

2 Onken SJ, Craig CM, Ridgway P, Ralph RO, Cook JA: An analysis of the definitions and elements of recovery: a review of the literature. Psych Rehabil J 2007; 31:9–22.

3 Harvey PD, Bellack AS: Toward a terminology for functional recovery in schizophrenia: is functional remission a viable concept? Schizophr Bull 2009;35: 300–306.

4 Lieberman JA, Drake RE, Sederer LL, Belger A, Keefe R, Perkins D, Stroup S: Science and Recovery in Schizophrenia. Psychiatr Serv 2008;59:487–496.

5 McGurk SR, Mueser KT, DeRosa TJ, Wolfe R: Work, recovery, and comorbidity in schizophrenia: a randomized controlled trial of cognitive remediation. Schizophr Bull 2009:35:319–335.

6 Bellack AS: Scientific and consumer models of recovery in schizophrenia: concordance, contrasts, and implications. Schizophr Bull 2006;32:432–442.

7 Davidson L, Roe D: Recovery from versus recovery in serious mental illness: one strategy for lessening confusion plaguing recovery. J Ment Health 2007;16: 459–470.

8 Lieberman RP, Kopelowicz A: Recovery from schizophrenia: a concept in search of research. Psychiatr Serv 2005;56:735–742.

9 Green MF, Kern RS, Braff DL, Mintz J: Neurocognitive deficits and functional outcome in schizophrenia: are we measuring the 'right stuff?' Schizophr Bull 2000;26:119–136.

10 Mausbach BT, Moore R, Bowie C, Cardenas V, Patterson TL: A review of instruments for measuring functional recovery in those diagnosed with psychosis. Schizophr Bull 2009:35307–35318.

11 Horan WP, Kring AM, Blanchard JJ: Anhedonia in schizophrenia: a review of assessment strategies. Schizophr Bull 2005;32:259–273.

12 Deegan PE: Recovery as a journey of the heart. Psychiatr Rehabil J 1996;19:91–97.

13 Brekke JS, Phillips E, Pancake L, Oh A, Lewis J, Duke J: Implementation practice and implementation research: a report from the field. Res Soc Work Pract, in press.

14 Brekke J, Long J: Community-based psychosocial rehabilitation and prospective change in functional, clinical, and subjective experience variables in schizophrenia. Schizophr Bull 2000;26:667–680.

15 Hemsley DR: The development of a cognitive model of schizophrenia: placing it in context. Neurosci Biobehav Rev 2005;29:977–988.

16 Bell MD, Mishara AL: Does negative symptom change relate to neurocognitive change in schizophrenia? Implications for targeted treatments. Schizophr Res 2006;81:17–27.

17 Bowie CR, Reichenberg A, Patterson TL, Heaton RK, Harvey PD: Determinants of real-world functioning performance in schizophrenia: correlations with cognition, functional capacity, and symptoms. Am J Psychiatry 2006;163:418–425.

18 Green MF, Kern RS, Heaton RK: Longitudinal studies of cognition and functional outcome in schizophrenia: implication for MATRICSS. Schizophr Res 2004;72:41–51.

19 Murray CL, Lopez AD: The Global Burden of Disease. Cambridge, Harvard University Press, 1996.

20 Brekke J: Functional outcome assessment in schizophrenia (invited presentation to NIMH-sponsored conference Measurement and Treatment Research to Improve Cognition in Schizophrenia). Bethesda, April 14–15, 2003.

21 Green MF, Penn DL, Bentall R, Carpenter WT, Gaebel W, Gur RC, Kring AM, Park S: Social cognition in schizophrenia: an NIMH workshop on definitions, assessment, and research opportunities. Schizophr Bull 2008;34:1211–1220.

22 Harvey PD: Functional recovery in schizophrenia: raising the bar for outcomes in people with schizophrenia. Schizophr Bull 2009;35:299.

23 McKibbin CL, Brekke JS, Siresa D, Jeste DV, Patterson TL: Direct assessment of functional abilities: relevance to persons with schizophrenia. Schizophr Res 2004;72:53–67.

24 Bellack AS, Green MF, Cook JA, Fenton W, Harvey PD, Heaton RK, Laughren T, Leon AC, Mayo DJ, Patrick DL, Patterson TL, Rose A, Stover E, Wykes T: Assessment of community functioning in people with schizophrenia and other severe mental illness: a white paper based on an NIMH-sponsored workshop. Schizophr Bull 2007;33:805–822.

25 Harvey PD, Velligan DI, Bellack AS: Performance-based measures of functional skills: usefulness in clinical treatment studies. Schizophr Bull 2007;33: 1138–1148.

26 Green MF: What are the functional consequences of neurocognitive deficits in schizophrenia? Am J Psychiatry 1996;153:321–330.

27 Heinrichs RW, Zakzanis KK: Neurocognitive deficit in schizophrenia: a quantitative review of the evidence. Neuropsychology 1998;12:426–445.

28 Kurtz MM, Wexler BE, Fujimoto M, Shagan DS, Seltzer JC: Symptoms versus neurocognition as predictors of change in life skills in schizophrenia after outpatient rehabilitation. Schizophr Res 2008;102: 303–311.

29 Keefe RSE, Sweeney JA, Gu H, Hamer RM, Perkins DO, McEvoy JP, Lieberman JA: Effects of olanzapine, quetiapine, and risperidone on neurocognitive function in early psychosis : a randomized, double-blind 52-week comparison. Am J Psychiatry 2007; 164:1061–1071.

30 McGurk SR, Meltzer HY: The role of cognition in vocational functioning in schizophrenia. Schizophr Res 2000;45:175–184.

31 Addington J, Saeedi H, Addington D: The course of cognitive functioning in first episode psychosis: changes over time and impact on outcome. Schizophr Res 2005;78:35–43.

32 Brekke JS, Kay DD, Kee KS, Green MF: Biosocial pathways to functional outcome in schizophrenia. Schizophr Res 2005;80:213–225.

33 Brekke JS, Hoe M, Long J, Green MF: How neurocognition and social cognition influence functional change during community-based psychosocial rehabilitation for individuals with schizophrenia. Schizophr Bull 2007;33:1247–1256.

34 McGurk SR, Mueser KT: Cognitive functioning, symptoms, and work in supported employment: a review and heuristic model. Schizophr Res 2004; 70:147–173.

35 Kurtz MM, Moberg PJ, Gur RC, Gur RE: Approaches to cognitive remediation of neuropsychological deficits in schizophrenia: a review and meta-analysis. Neuropsychol Rev Publ 2001;11:197–210.

36 McGurk SR, Twamley EW, Sitzer DI, McHugo GJ, Mueser KT: A meta-analysis of cognitive remediation in schizophrenia. Am J Psychiatry 2007;164: 1791–1802.

37 Gold JM: Cognitive deficits as treatment targets in schizophrenia. Schizophr Res 2004;72:21–28.

38 Hogarty GE, Flesher S, Ulrich R, et al: Cognitive enhancement therapy for schizophrenia: effects of a two-year randomized trial on cognition and behavior. Arch Gen Psychiatry 2004;61:866–876.

39 McGurk SR, Mueser KT, Feldman K, Wolfe R, Pascaris A: Cognitive training for supported employment: 2–3 year outcomes of a randomized controlled trial. Am J Psychiatry 2007;164:437–441.

40 Roder V, Mueller DR, Mueser KT, Brenner HD: Integrated psychological therapy (IPT) for schizophrenia: is it effective? Schizophr Bull 2006;32(suppl 1):S81–S93.

41 Twamley EW, Jeste DV, Bellack AS: A review of cognitive training in schizophrenia. Schizophr Bull 2003; 29:359–382.

42 Sergi MJ, Rassovsky Y, Nuechterlein KH, Green MF: Social perception as a mediator of the influence of early visual processing on functional status in schizophrenia. Schizophr Res 2006;163:448–454.

43 Vauth R, Rusch N, Wirtz,M, Corrigan PW: Does social cognition influence the relation between neurocognitive deficits and vocational functioning in schizophrenia? Psychiatry Res 2004;128:155–165.

44 Adolphs R: Social cognition and the human brain. Trends Cogn Sci 1999;3:469–479.

45 Brothers L: The social brain: a project for integrating primate behavior and neurophysiology in a new domain. Concepts Neurosci 1990;1:27–51.

46 Couture SM, Penn DL, Roberts DL: The functional significance of social cognition in schizophrenia: a review. Schizophr Bull 2006;32:S44–S63.

47 Penn DL, Sanna LJ, Roberts DL: Social cognition in schizophrenia: an overview. Schizophr Bull 2008; 34:408–411.

48 Pinkham AE, Hopfinger JB, Pelphrey KA, Pivenc J, Penn DL: Neural bases for impaired social cognition in schizophrenia and autism spectrum disorders. Schizophr Res 2008;99:164–175.

49 Kohler CG, Brennan AR: Recognition of facial emotions in schizophrenia. Curr Opin Psychiatry 2004; 17:81–86.

50 Mandal MK, Pandey R, Prasad AB: Facial expressions of emotion and schizophrenia: a review. Schizophr Bull 1998;24:399–412.

51 Green MJ. Phillips ML: Social threat perception and the evolution of paranoia. Neurosci Biobehav Rev 2004;28:333–342.

52 Penn DL, Ritchie M, Francis J, Combs D, Martin J: Social perception in schizophrenia: the role of context. Psychiatry Res 2002;109:149–159.

53 Kim J, Doop ML, Blake R, Park S: Impaired visual recognition of biological motion in schizophrenia. Schizophr Res 2005;77:299–307.

54 Hooker C, Park S: Emotion processing and its relationship to social functioning in schizophrenia patients. Psychiatry Res 2002;112:41–50.

55 Kee KS, Green MF, Mintz J, Brekke JS: Is emotional processing a predictor of functional outcome in schizophrenia? Schizophr Bull 2003;29:487–497.

56 Brune M: 'Theory of mind in schizophrenia: a review of the literature. Schizophr Bull 2005;31:21–42.

57 Lysaker PH, Lancaster RS, Nees MA, Davis LW: Attributional style and symptoms as predictors of social function in schizophrenia. J Rehabil Res Dev 2004;41:225–232.

58 Brekke J: The relationship between cognitive and environmental determinants of the functional dimensions in schizophrenia. Invited presentation to NIMH-sponsored conference, Measurement and Treatment Research to Improve Cognition in Schizophrenia (MATRICS-CT). Bethesda, August 21–22, 2007.

59 Brekke JS, Kohrt B Green MF: Neuropsychological functioning as a moderator of the relationship between psychosocial functioning and the subjective experience of self and life in schizophrenia. Schizophr Bull 2001;27:697–708.

60 Barch DM: The Relationships among cognition, motivation, and emotion in schizophrenia: how much and how little we know. Schizophr Bull 2005; 31:875–881.

61 Velligan DI, Kern RS, Gold JM: Cognitive rehabilitation for schizophrenia and the putative role of motivation and expectancies. Schizophr Bull 2006;32: 474–485.

62 Measurement and Treatment Research to Improve Cognition in Schizophrenia, MATRICS. Maryland, New Approaches to Cognition Conference, Sept. 9–10, 2004.

63 Yamada A-M, Lee KH, Dinh TQ, Barrio C, Brekke JS: Intrinsic motivation as a mediator of relationships between symptoms and functioning among individuals with schizophrenia-spectrum disorders in a diverse urban community. J Nerv Ment Dis, in press.

64 Braitman A, Counts P, Davenport R, Zurlinden B, Rogers M, Clauss J, Kulkarni A, Kymla J, Montgomery I: Comparison of barriers to employment for unemployed and employed clients in a case management program: an exploratory study. Psychiatr Rehabil J 1995;19:3–8.

65 Penn DL, Combs D: Modification of affect perception deficits in schizophrenia. Schizophr Res 2000; 46:217–229.

66 Schmand B, Kuipers T, Van der Gaag M, Bosveld J, Bulthuis F, Jellema M: Cognitive disorders and negative symptoms as correlates of motivational deficits in psychotic patients. Psychol Med 1994;24:869–884.

67 Summerfelt AT, Alphs LD, Wagman AM, Funderburk FR, Hierholzer RM, Strauss ME: Reduction of perseverative errors in patients with schizophrenia using monetary feedback. J Abnorm Psychol 1991;100:613–616.

68 Medalia, A, Choi J: Cognitive remediation in schizophrenia. Neuropsychol Rev DOI: 10.1007/s11065-009-9097-y.

69 Nakagami E, Xie B, Hoe M, Brekke JS: Intrinsic motivation, neurocognition and psychosocial functioning in schizophrenia: testing mediator and moderator effects. Schizophr Res 2008;105:95–104.

70 Sharma T, Antova L: Cognitive function in schizophrenia: deficits, functional consequences, and future treatment. Psychiatr Clin North Am 2003;26: 25–40.

71 Heggestad E, Kanfer R: Individual differences in trait motivation: development of the Motivational Trait Questionnaire (MTQ). Int J Educ Res 2000;33: 751–776.

72 Barch DM: Emotion, motivation, and reward processing in schizophrenia spectrum disorders: what we know and where we need to go. Schizophr Bull 2008;34:816–818.

73 Horvath AO: The therapeutic alliance: concepts, research and training. Aust Psychologist 2001;36: 170–176.

74 Davis LW, Lysaker PH: Therapeutic alliance and improvements in work performance over time in patients with schizophrenia. J Nerv Ment Dis 2007; 195:353–357.

75 Addington J, Addington D: Neurocognitive and social functioning in schizophrenia. Schizophr Bull 1999;25:173–182.

John S. Brekke, PhD
School of Social Work, MC-0411, University of Southern California
Los Angeles, CA 90089–0411 (USA)
Tel. +1 213 740 0297, E-Mail brekke@usc.edu

Roder V, Medalia A (eds): Neurocognition and Social Cognition in Schizophrenia Patients. Basic Concepts and Treatment. Key Issues Ment Health. Basel, Karger, 2010, vol 177, pp 37–49

3

Treatment Approaches with a Special Focus on Neurocognition: Overview and Empirical Results

Matthew M. Kurtz[a] · Gudrun Sartory[b]

[a]Department of Psychology, Wesleyan University, Middletown, Conn., USA; [b]Department of Psychology, University of Wuppertal, Wuppertal, Germany

Abstract

Research on neuropsychological interventions designed to help reduce the functional consequences of impairments in elementary neurocognitive function (e.g. attention, memory and problem-solving), collectively labeled cognitive remediation for individuals with schizophrenia, is critically synthesized. Methods for remediation of deficits in neurocognition in schizophrenia are organized and discussed in terms of computer-assisted versus clinician-guided approaches and individualized versus group approaches. The results revealed that a wide array of interventions, diverse in terms of focus (drill-and-practice training in elementary neurocognitive skills versus acquisition of strategies for bypassing neurocognitive deficits), and whether cognitive training was offered as an isolated treatment or embedded as part of more complex social skill training programs, produced improvements on neurocognitive measures distinct from those trained. Potential mechanisms of improvement in studies of remediation, as well as the evidence for the generalization of improvements to a variety of indices of more global psychosocial function are discussed. Several directions for future research are proposed.

Copyright © 2010 S. Karger AG, Basel

The goals of this chapter are to (1) offer a brief history of the development of cognitive remediation interventions for individuals with schizophrenia by highlighting 2 of the seminal studies in this area; (2) synthesize findings from a variety of individualized approaches to the remediation of neurocognitive deficits, including computer-assisted and therapist-guided approaches; (3) provide a critical synthesis of 4 quantitative meta-analyses that have been conducted on individualized approaches to cognitive remediation, and (4) review the current status of group-based approaches to cognitive remediation. Our chapter is restricted to the review of training programs for acquiring skills to improve elementary cognitive function directly, rather than interventions targeted at modifying environments to enhance psychosocial function.

Brief History of Cognitive Remediation

Any overview of the history of the study of cognitive rehabilitation interventions in schizophrenia would be remiss in failing to include 2 highly influential early papers by Wagner [1] and Meichenbaum and Cameron [2] that supported the utility of 2 very different behavioral interventions for improving performance on measures of neurocognition. These studies are particularly important in that they emphasize 2 very different approaches to the rehabilitation of cognitive deficits that continue to characterize the field today: on the one hand, the repeated practice of elementary neurocognitive tasks as a means of strengthening underfunctioning information processing mechanisms (and presumably underlying neural systems) in the context of gradually increasing task difficulty, and on the other hand, the teaching of strategies that are not task specific and are designed to be employed in a variety of life settings, that help compensate for persistent deficits in elementary neurocognition and that would be expected to promote generalization from the training environment to everyday life.

As a very early example of the drill-and-practice approach, Wagner [1] investigated the effects of contingent reinforcement and repeated practice on a delayed matching-to-sample training task, on a variety of neuropsychological outcome measures in individuals with schizophrenia. The outcome measures included the similarities subtest of the Wechsler Adult Intelligence Scale, Proverbs Test, Memory for Designs Test, Letter Circle Test and the Peabody Picture Vocabulary Test. These tests were administered at a pretraining baseline and after 4 days of training. The performance in remediated subjects improved on 4 out of the 5 tasks relative to contact and no-contact control groups. The strengths of the study included carefully selected control groups that addressed the effects of exposure to the experimenter, contact with the training apparatus and noncontingent reinforcement.

Meichenbaum and Cameron [2] investigated the effects of a self-instructional (SI) training procedure in altering the attention, thinking and language behaviors of hospitalized participants with schizophrenia. In experiment 1 participants were taught to (a) verbalize the nature and demands of the task; (b) practice cognitive rehearsal and planning to help maintain task focus; (c) give self-instructions in the form of self-guidance; (d) give coping self-statement to handle failure and frustration, and (e) provide self-reinforcement to maintain task perseverance. The results showed significant improvements in performance on a digit recall and a digit symbol task relative to control groups that received either no treatment or met with the experimenters and practiced tests but did not receive specific SI training. In experiment 2, an expanded SI training procedure was used to include covert rehearsal for social interactions. A wider range of dependent variables was assessed. The results indicated that SI training: (1) produced stronger digit recall performance under conditions of distraction; (2) produced more abstract interpretations of proverbs in patients, and (3) reduced the number of irrelevant verbalizations to interview questions. The strengths of these experiments included the practice and nonpractice control groups and the range of dependent measures that were evaluated. Limitations were thelarge effort required to teach such highly sophisticated cognitive training techniques. The authors concluded that this process of instruction produced substantive gains in elementary cognitive functioning as well as enhanced social skill.

Forms of Training

A variety of methods have been employed in neurocognitive training. They comprise remediation exercises administered to individuals or groups, paper-and-pencil tasks, computer-assisted tasks or procedural learning training such as learning to assemble an object. Finally, they may convey a strategy with which to approach a task or merely consist of rote learning.

Computer-Assisted Approaches

Typically under the supervision of a clinician, patients are given computerized tasks which target particular cognitive functions and are usually designed to be adaptive, i.e. increase in difficulty according to the patient's performance. There are a number of such programs available. An example of a commonly used program is Cogpack [3], with tasks aimed at improving a variety of cognitive domains such as attention and concentration, psychomotor speed, learning and memory as well as executive functions. Participants are given feedback on their performance following completion of each exercise. The tasks were designed to be enjoyable and reinforcing to complete, frequently depicting everyday events. For instance, a visual memory task shows a city street with moving vehicles, people and stores. The scene is shown for several seconds and participants are then asked to recall details of the scene.

An early study suggested that computerized training of attention and short-term memory has a beneficial effect on reaction time in a modality shift paradigm [4], and 18 sessions of computerized training yielded a significant improvement with regard to the Continuous Performance Test [5]. On the other hand, although the performance on a computer-mediated vigilance task improved over time, this gain failed to generalize to other cognitive tasks [6]. Neurocognitive enhancement therapy including computer-based training on attention, memory and executive function, together with work therapy, resulted in a superior outcome in terms of working memory and executive function as compared to work therapy only [7, 8]. The effects endured for up to 6 months after training [9]. Massed practice of Cogpack training in inpatients, i.e. 15 sessions within 3 weeks, resulted in improvement of episodic verbal learning and executive function compared to a wait list control group [10]. Computer-assisted remediation raining also had a better outcome than an enriched supportive therapy condition [11]. Finally, processing speed as measured with the digit symbol test was also found to increase with computer-mediated training [11, 12]. There is little evidence to date for improvement in visual learning and memory [13]. Thus, while there have been some exceptions, the balance of studies in this domain has reported positive results of cognitive remediation on neurocognitive measures that are distinct from those trained, despite wide differences in sample characteristics, methodological approach and neurocognitive outcome measures selected [see 123].

Little is known as yet about the mechanisms mediating neurocognitive improvement as a result of individualized, computer-assisted training. The underlying assumption of the majority of these studies is that repeated practice strengthens the targeted neurocognitive skill directly. The possibility can, however, not be ruled out that compensatory strategies are acquired or that the stimulating training has a general and nonspecific activating effect on cognitive functions. In an attempt to unravel some of the underlying mechanisms, Kurtz et al. [12] carried out a dismantling study comparing targeted computer-assisted remediation training with training in the use of computers, i.e. computer literacy. The latter also conveyed a skill and provided cognitive enrichment, albeit nonspecific. The results revealed that cognitive remediation training produced significant enhancement in working memory but both groups showed overall improvements in reasoning/executive function, verbal and spatial episodic memory, and processing speed. It is conceivable that different cognitive functions respond in distinct ways to different remediation strategies.

Clinician-Guided Approaches

Among studies of cognitive training that are clinician guided, without the aid of a computer, attention and working memory were repeatedly found to improve [14, 15], as did measures of emotion perception and executive function [e.g. 15]. The improvements could be shown to be durable [16], indicative of the continued use of the acquired skills by the patients.

A number of different remediation techniques have been used in clinician-guided cognitive remediation, some of which have been applied previously in patients with neurocognitive disorders due to brain injury. Given the schizophrenia patients' deficits in short-term memory, errorless learning was an obvious candidate. The technique was originally designed to prevent patients from storing errors they made rather than the correct information. There are 4 components to this technique: (a) the tasks to be learned are broken down in their components starting with the most basic units; (b) training starts with the simplest task and (c) progresses step-wise to the more difficult ones, and (d) performance of each step is overlearned while probands are given verbal instructions (so that errors do not occur) and abundant positive reinforcement. Kern et al. [17] found the technique to be useful for the acquisition of new skills in patients. Wykes et al. [14] also stressed the importance of immediate feedback and reinforcement upon the successful completion of a task as well as massed practice.

In schizophrenia remediation studies, errorless learning has often been implemented in a manualized cognitive skills program [18] which consists of 40 face-to-face sessions, using paper-and-pencil exercises and aimed at the teaching of strategic information processing. Therapy is individualized and there is support for the cognitive gains to be transferred to the real world. Three cognitive domains are targeted, cognitive flexibility, working memory and planning. Each of the modules consists of a series of tasks starting from an 'extremely easy' to an 'easy' level of difficulty. The cognitive flexibility module requires patients to engage, disengage and re-engage attention to a particular cognitive set or between sets. In the working memory module, they are given practice in maintaining 2 sets of information simultaneously and to carry out transformations on a held information set. Finally, the planning module consists of tasks in which sequences of moves have to be planned for the participants to reach certain goals. To attain them, the provided information needs to be organized and subgoals determined. Furthermore, emphasis is placed upon the use of these strategies in everyday life, for example when going shopping. Participants are encouraged to reflect themselves on how these strategies might be implemented in everyday activities. The program produced durable improvements in working memory [19] as well as some progress in cognitive flexibility. The improvement in working memory was predictive of those in social functioning.

Further techniques are the use of procedural or motor learning strategies, the latter of which is not as impaired as verbal learning in schizophrenia. 'Chunking' information, i.e. breaking information down in separate units, or categorizing information are further strategies to facilitate processing and learning new information. The technique of scaffolding [20] provides learning support for tasks that are arranged to increase only slightly in difficulty over time. Finally, attention shaping was conceived to improve attentiveness and learning of social skills in schizophrenia patients [21]. The shaping technique targets a particular behavior and selectively reinforces its stepwise increment. In the study by Silverstein et al. [21] patients were rewarded for increasing attentiveness during training of social skills in a group. The results of this study not only showed that patients with attention shaping demonstrated more attentiveness in the group sessions than the mere social skills training condition, but increased attentiveness was also related to a higher level of social skill acquisition. An instrumental learning procedure could thus be shown to improve cognitive and behavioral functions.

Meta-Analyses

To date, 5 quantitative meta-analyses have been published, focused almost exclusively on individualized approaches to neurocognitive remediation for schizophrenia. The first meta-analytic investigation by Kurtz et al. [22], compiled results from a variety of methods of training on the Wisconsin Card Sorting Test (WCST), a measure of rule-learning and conceptual flexibility, on several dependent measures from the task in individuals with schizophrenia. WCST training studies were selected for analysis as they represented the largest body of research into interventions targeted at a consistent neurocognitive outcome measure in the extant literature at the time of the review. Interest in the modification of performance on the WCST grew out of speculation that impairment on this task was a reflection of a static, structural damage to the dorsolateral prefrontal cortex in individuals diagnosed as having schizophrenia. Work in this area was spurred by an initial study by Goldberg et al. [23], who reported in a sample of 44 long-term inpatients that the performance on the WCST could not be improved by offering information on the nature of the categories in the task, the occurrence of shifts in set and card-by-card instruction in how to do the task. The authors concluded that impairment on the WCST in schizophrenia reflected a stable deficit, likely linked to static, dorsolateral prefrontal cortex dysfunction.

In response to these negative findings, along with their potential treatment implications, a number of laboratories ran similar studies evaluating a variety of methods of training on the WCST. The instructional techniques employed in these studies included task explanations and card-by-card instructions similar to those utilized by Goldberg et al. [23], errorless learning methods, in which the WCST is broken down into smaller elements and each element is trained individually with minimal opportunity for error commission, and self-monitoring interventions in which the participants are simply asked to verbalize their sorting strategy on the WCST. The meta-analytic results of these studies revealed mean weighted effect sizes for categories achieved, perseverative errors and conceptual level responses from the WCST all in the large range (Cohen's d effect-sizes = 1.08, 0.93 and 0.90, respectively). There was no evidence for heterogeneity in the analysis, suggesting that the effects were consistent despite the diverse array of training strategies employed. The limitations of the analysis included the focus on brevity (typically 1-session interventions), inclusion of studies that trained and tested on the same neurocognitive measure, and lack of assessment of generalization of training effects to other measures of cognition and function.

Pilling et al. [24], in the second meta-analysis of remediation studies, came to quite different conclusions regarding the value of cognitive remediation strategies for improving neurocognitive function in schizophrenia. The inclusion criteria for their meta-analysis were a randomized, controlled study design, restriction of the study sample to individuals with schizophrenia, and an explicit goal of treatment for improving cognitive skills, using procedures intended to improve the level of a specified cognitive skill. A total of 5 studies of 170 participants met their criteria for inclusion and presented usable data. The results revealed no benefits of cognitive remediation on attention, verbal memory, visual memory and symptoms when compared to the control conditions. The authors concluded that there was little justification from their analysis to include cognitive training interventions as a component of rehabilitation interventions for individuals diagnosed as having schizophrenia. The tiny number of studies included in this meta-analysis, however, raises questions regarding the meaningfulness of the reported conclusions. In addition, a variety of randomized, controlled remediation studies that met criteria for inclusion in their paper [e.g. 20] were overlooked in this review, also making conclusions tenuous.

Krabbendam and Aleman [25] conducted a meta-analysis of all studies of cognitive remediation that were (a) randomized trials with a control condition (within- or between-group), (b) not limited to training on a single cognitive task, and (c) had training methods different from the assessment measures. A total of 12 studies met the criteria. Effect sizes were measured as a change from before to after treatment in the experimental condition, as compared to change in the control condition. When multiple measures of cognitive function were administered in a single study, these values were averaged to calculate a composite cognition score for the study. The mean weighted effect size was 0.45 for cognitive measures. Moderator analyses did not reveal effects of number of training sessions on the size of the training effects. There was some evidence for superior effects of strategy-based training on cognitive outcome measures relative to restorative approaches.

Twamley et al. [26], in a review and meta-analysis of 17 studies of cognitive training in schizophrenia, categorized interventions as to their location on a continuum from largely strategy-based to involving automated repetition, and whether they were computer assisted or not. Studies that utilized outcome measures identical to measures that were trained were excluded from the review, as were brief, laboratory-administered interventions for improving cognition (e.g. increasing stimulus duration on a sustained attention test). One study, focused on environmental modifications for bypassing cognitive deficits, was considered separately. The results from this analysis revealed weighted mean effect sizes of 0.32 for measures of neurocognition, 0.26 for reductions in symptom severity and a 0.51 effect size improvement in everyday functioning. With the exception of computer-assisted strategy training, computer-assisted and non-computer-assisted approaches, and both interventions based on strategy and automated repetition were shown to produce positive results. The small number of studies, their small sample sizes, the failure to correct for multiple comparisons and the especially limited number of studies assessing generalization of remediation effects to symptoms and everyday outcome were noted.

In the most comprehensive and up-to-date meta-analytic investigation, McGurk et al. [13] evaluated 26 randomized, controlled studies consisting of 1,151 individuals with schizophrenia and found a significant effect size of 0.41 for cognitive function with a durability of effects of 0.66, a slightly smaller effect of 0.36 for psychosocial function and a small but significant effect for symptoms at 0.28. For findings on cognitive outcome measures, the effect sizes differed with regard to different domains,

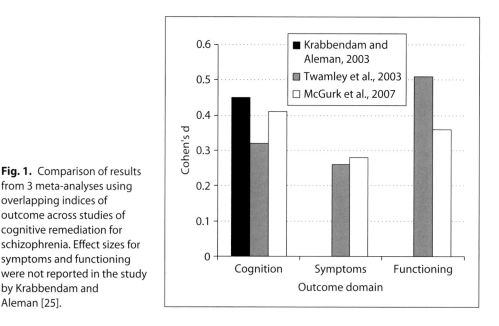

Fig. 1. Comparison of results from 3 meta-analyses using overlapping indices of outcome across studies of cognitive remediation for schizophrenia. Effect sizes for symptoms and functioning were not reported in the study by Krabbendam and Aleman [25].

with the highest benefits conveyed on social cognition, verbal working memory and processing speed. These are also the functions which received most training. Drill-and-practice remediation efforts as well as more hours of therapy produced larger effects on verbal memory. For psychosocial function, the effects were markedly larger in studies where cognitive training was offered as a component of a more comprehensive rehabilitation intervention. The effects on psychosocial function were also larger for studies using drill-and-practice and strategy coaching as compared to drill-and-practice alone, and older versus younger patients. A summary of results from meta-analyses utilizing comparable outcome measures discussed in this section is presented in figure 1.

Since this last meta-analysis, a number of additional remediation studies have been carried out, which were summarized by Wykes and Huddy [27]. These more recent studies vary in terms of rehabilitation paradigms and employed techniques and thus also fail to produce a unified outcome. However, the authors also conclude that cognitive change can be induced by cognitive training in schizophrenia and that it has a more wide-spread effect when combined with other approaches such as vocational training. Finally, they noted that cognitive training is valued by the patients, which is reflected in improvements of self-esteem and quality of life.

In conclusion, 5 meta-analyses on cognitive remediation in schizophrenia have revealed (1) moderate size effects of training on cognition; (2) moderate size effects of training on psychosocial function; (3) some evidence that effects on psychosocial function emerge only when cognitive remediation is offered as part of a more comprehensive rehabilitation intervention, and (4) little evidence to date that the duration of the remediation treatment has measurable effects on most domains of response. Meta-analyses to date have informed us little about which clients are most likely to benefit from these interventions and which methods of intervention (computer-assisted vs. non-computer-assisted, strategy-based vs. drill-and-practice) are likely to yield the largest treatment effects.

Group Approaches to Cognitive Rehabilitation

The most well-studied group approach to cognitive rehabilitation interventions is integrated psychological therapy, or IPT, as developed and studied by Brenner, Roder et al. [28] in Europe, as well as Spaulding et al. [29] at the University of Nebraska among others. IPT is described in detail in another chapter and thus is only briefly described here. The results from studies of IPT have been very promising. A recent meta-analysis including 29 randomized, controlled studies of IPT yielded several interesting findings. The effect sizes for measures of neurocognition were in the moderate to large size (0.61), and importantly effects were also evident, albeit in a slightly attenuated form, on measures of psychosocial functioning (0.41). In considering IPT as a group format for cognitive remediation, it remains unclear what the mechanisms of treatment effects are, as training in cognitive remediation is included with training of social skills. To address this issue, Spaulding et al. [28] investigated the effectiveness of the 3 cognitive subcomponents of IPT (cognitive differentiation, social perception and verbal communication) against a supportive therapy condition matched for clinician contact, and duration and frequency of the sessions, in a sample of 90 hospitalized patients with severe and persistent mental illness. All patients participated in an enriched and comprehensive set of psychiatric rehabilitation interventions in addition to their experimental or control treatment. The results revealed improvement on a measure of attention and a performance-based measure of problem-solving in the experimental condition, relative to the control condition, with improvement evident in both conditions on measures of attention, memory and executive function. These data suggest that IPT effects on cognition are mediated, at least in part, by training of cognitive skills in the first 3, cognitively focused modules of the program. The findings also point to large, nonspecific effects of rehabilitation interventions on elementary neurocognitive function.

An exciting new development in technologies for group treatment of cognitive deficits in individuals diagnosed as having schizophrenia is the use of group interventions targeted specifically at the acquisition of an array of compensatory strategies for helping clients circumvent their cognitive difficulties. In contrast to studies of drill-and-practice elementary neurocognitive training, these approaches emphasize bypassing cognitive deficits through strategies and, similar to IPT, linking these strategies tightly with everyday life activities to promote generalization. Twamley et al. [30] have developed a manualized intervention consisting of a series of modules in which both internal (use of acronyms and visual imagery) and external supports (writing down lists, placing lists in a convenient and visible location on the home environment) are utilized to support a variety of instrumental everyday life skills identified as important by both consumers, their family members and health-care professionals. These skills are grouped into 4 general domains of prospective memory, attention and vigilance, learning and memory, and executive function that are taught sequentially. Examples of everyday tasks include remembering to go to work or school (prospective memory unit), maintaining attention in class (attention and vigilance), learning and remembering names of supervisors (learning and memory) and self-monitoring performance at work (executive function). Pilot testing has indicated that this intervention produces medium effect size improvement on verbal learning and executive function measures, and large effect size improvement in passive auditory attention at a 6-month follow-up after cessation of treatment. Preliminary findings also indicate generalization of effects to such treatment-resistant facets of the illness as negative symptoms and quality of life.

Conclusions

To date, a panoply of cognitive interventions have been developed to address elementary deficits in neurocognition that differ in terms of whether they are (1) conducted in an individualized format or in a group; (2) conducted with a computer or therapist-guided, and (3) administered along with treatment targeted at more complex aspects of social skill (IPT). The results have revealed strong support for moderate (approximately 0.4 SD) [13] improvements on measures of neurocognitive function distinct from the tasks trained as part of specific remediation protocols. These findings are important in that they suggest that these training protocols are producing improvement in the underlying neurocognitive skill necessary to successfully complete neurocognitive tasks, rather than teaching skills to the specific test. These findings are also remarkable given the wide differences in patient sample composition, method of remediation, and duration and intensity of intervention administration in studies in this research area. We note that the specificity of these reported effects remains unclear. Two studies [12, 29] in which cognitive remediation interventions were compared to tightly matched control conditions including similar levels of supportive clinician contact, and in which study patients were administered an array of rehabilitation services, produced large effects on neurocognitive measures in the absence of specific remediation interventions. Other studies, however, that have compared effects of cognitive remediation to control conditions consisting of active rehabilitation interventions such as supported employment or work therapy [6] have not shown these types of nonspecific effects.

A major limitation of the work to date in remediation in schizophrenia is the paucity of studies assessing the generalization of cognitive training effects to outcome

Cognitive remediation training tasks →	Elementary neurocognitive measures distinct from training tasks →	Social cognitive measures (e.g., facial affect recognition, theory-of-mind and attributional bias) →	Performance-based measures of interpersonal and daily living skill. →	Psychosocial function measures and negative symptoms
Proximal	———————————	———————————	——————————→	Distal
		Outcome measures		

Fig. 2. A proposed organization for outcome measures in studies of cognitive rehabilitation in schizophrenia. Larger effects are presumed for outcome measures more proximal to the site of the intervention.

measures distal from the locus of the remediation intervention. In the meta-analysis by McGurk et al. [13] only 11 randomized, controlled remediation studies included functional outcome measures, and these measures varied widely in terms of whether they were clinician-rated, performance-based (based on a laboratory assessment of life or social skills) or global ratings of function. It seems highly unlikely that cognitive remediation interventions would produce equivalent effects on such a variety of outcome measures that have uncertain relationships to neurocognitive functioning. To enhance our understanding of the mechanisms of action of remediation interventions, future studies could benefit from utilizing a variety of outcome measures that vary systematically in terms of their putative proximity to the site of the remediation intervention. An example of a classification system of outcome measures is presented in figure 2.

As can be seen, in this model, performance-based measures of everyday life and social skill that are administered in a laboratory, could be viewed as intermediary measures, less influenced by cognitive interventions than standardized neuropsychological measures but more likely to show treatment effects than clinician-rated measures of community function or negative symptoms, which are likely to be influenced by a broader array of social factors. Importantly, this model does not include measures of self-reported life satisfaction and self-esteem as treatment endpoints, as the relationship between these measures, and changes in performance-based and clinician-rated measures of functional status after rehabilitation interventions remain unclear and even paradoxical in some studies. The effects of cognitive remediation on self-reported quality of life remain largely unknown and should be an important focus of future studies.

References

1 Wagner BR: The training of attending and abstracting responses in chronic schizophrenics. J Exp Res Personality 1968;3:77–88.

2 Meichenbaum D, Cameron R: Training schizophrenics to talk to themselves: a means of developing attention controls. Behav Ther 1973;4:515–534.

3 COGPACK. Marker Software. Ladenburg. http://www.cogpack.com/USA/frames.htm.

4 Hermanutz M, Gestrich J: Computer-assisted attention training in schizophrenics: a comparative study. Eur Arch Psychiatry Clin Neurosci 1991;240:282–287.

5 Medalia A, Aluma M, Tryon W, Merriam AE: Effectiveness of attention training in schizophrenia. Schizophr Bull 1998;24:147–152.

6 Benedict RHB, Harris AE, Markow T, McCormick JA, Nuechterlein KH, Asarnow RF: Effects of attention training on information processing in schizophrenia. Schizophr Bull 1994;20:537–546.

7 Bell M, Bryson G, Graig T, Corcoran C, Wexler BE: Neurocognitive enhancement therapy with work therapy. Arch Gen Psychiatry 2001;58:763–768.

8 Greig TC, Zito W, Wexler BE, Fiszdon J, Bell MD: Improved cognitive function in schizophrenia after one year of cognitive training and vocational services. Schizophr Res 2007;96:156–161.

9 Bell M, Bryson G, Wexler BE: Cognitive remediation of working memory deficits: durability of training effects in severely impaired and less severely impaired schizophrenia. Acta Psychiatr Scand 2003; 108:101–109.

10 Sartory G, Zorn C, Groetzinger G, Windgassen K: Computerized cognitive remediation improves verbal learning and processing speed in schizophrenia. Schizophr Res 2005;75:219–223.

11 Hogarty GE, Flesher S, Ulrich R, Carter M, Greenwald D, Pogue-Geile M, Kechavan M, Cooley S, DiBarry AL, Garrett A, Parepally H, Zoretich R: Cognitive enhancement therapy for schizophrenia: effects of a 2-year randomized trial on cognition and behaviour. Arch Gen Psychiatry 2004;61:866–876.

12 Kurtz MM, Seltzer JC, Shagan DS, Thime WR, Wexler BE: Computer-assisted cognitive remediation in schizophrenia: what is the active ingredient? Schizophr Res 2007;89:251–260.

13 McGurk SR, Twamley EW, Sitzer DI, McHugo GJ, Mueser KT: A meta-analysis of cognitive remediation in schizophrenia. Am J Psychiatry 2007;164:1791–1802.

14 Wykes T, Reeder C, Corner J, Williams C, Everitt B: The effects of neurocognitive remediation on executive processing in patients with schizophrenia. Schizophr Bull 1999;28:291–307.

15 Van der Gaag M, Kern RS, von den Bosch RJ, Liberman RP: A controlled trial of cognitive remediation in schizophrenia. Schizophr Bull 2002;28: 167–176.

16 Wykes T, Reeder C, Corner J, Rice C, Williams C, Everitt B: Are the effects of cognitive remediation therapy (CRT) durable? Results from an exploratory trial in schizophrenia. Schizophr Bull 2003;61:163–174.

17 Kern RS, Green MF, Mintz J, Liberman RP: Does 'errorless learning' compensate for neurocognitive impairments in the work rehabilitation of persons with schizophrenia? Psychol Med 2003;33:433–442.

18 Delahunty A, Reeder C, Wykes T, et al: Revised Cognitive Remediation Therapy Manual. London, Institute of Psychiatry, 2002.

19 Wykes T, Reeder C, Landau S, Everitt B, Knapp M, Patel A, Romeo R: Cognitive remediation therapy in schizophrenia. Br J Psychiatry 2007;190:421–427.

20 Young DA, Freyslinger MG: Scaffolding instruction and the remediation of Wisconsin card sorting test deficits in chronic schizophrenia. Schizophr Res 1995;16:199–207.

21 Silverstein SM, Spaulding WD, Menditto AA, Savitz A, Liberman RP, Berten S, Starobin H: Attention shaping: a reward-based learning method to enhance skills training outcomes in schizophrenia. Schizophr Bull 2009;35:222–232.

22 Kurtz MM, Moberg PJ, Gur RC, Gur RE: Approaches to remediation of neuropsychological deficits in schizophrenia: a review and meta-analysis. Neuropsychol Rev 2001;1:197–210.

23 Goldberg TE, Weinberger, DR, Berman KF, Pliskin NH, Podd MH: Further evidence for dementia of the prefrontal type? Arch Gen Psychiatry 1987; 44:1008–1014.

24 Pilling S, Bebbington P, Kuipers E, Garety P, Geddes J, Orbach G, Morgan C: Psychological treatments in schizophrenia. II. Meta-analyses of randomized controlled trials of social skills training and cognitive remediation. Psychol Med 2002;32:783–791.

25 Krabbendam L, Aleman A: Cognitive rehabilitation in schizophrenia: a quantitative analysis of controlled trials. Psychopharmacology 2003;169:376–382.

26 Twamley EW, Jeste DV, Bellack AS: A review of cognitive training in schizophrenia. Schizophr Bull 2003;29:359–382.

27 Wykes T, Huddy V: Cognitive remediation for schizophrenia: it is even more complicated. Curr Opin Psychiatry 2009;22:161–167.

28 Roder V, Mueller DR, Muser KT, Brenner HD: Integrated psychological therapy (IPT) for schizophrenia: is it effective? Schizophr Bull 2006;32:S81–S93.

29 Spaulding WD, Reed D, Sullivan M, Richardson C, Weiler, M: Effects of cognitive treatment in psychiatric rehabilitation. Schizophr Bull 1999;25:657–676.

30 Twamley EW, Salva GH, Zurhellen CH, Heaton RK, Jeste DV: Development and pilot testing of a novel compensatory cognitive training intervention for people with psychosis. Am J Psychiatr Rehabil 2008;11:144–163.

Matthew M. Kurtz, PhD
Department of Psychology, Wesleyan University
207 High Street
Middletown, CT 06459 (USA)
Tel. +1 860 685 2072, Fax +1 860 685 2761, E-Mail mkurtz@wesleyan.edu

Roder V, Medalia A (eds): Neurocognition and Social Cognition in Schizophrenia Patients. Basic Concepts and Treatment. Key Issues Ment Health. Basel, Karger, 2010, vol 177, pp 50–60

3.1

Compensatory Cognitive Training

Elizabeth W. Twamley · Cynthia H. Zurhellen · Lea Vella

Department of Psychiatry, University of California, San Diego, Calif., USA

Abstract

As cognitive deficits are common in individuals with schizophrenia, attempts to remediate them are an important part of complete mental health interventions in this population. Cognitive training approaches may involve environmental modification, restoration and compensation. The cognitive training approach described in this chapter is a combination of both compensatory strategy training and client-driven environmental modification. In this manualized, group-based intervention, clients are introduced to strategies targeting the domains of prospective memory, attention and vigilance, learning and memory, and executive functioning. They then receive assistance in planning how to use the strategies in their everyday lives. Preliminary results from the current randomized controlled trial of this cognitive training intervention have shown promising results. Those who received the intervention showed medium to large positive effects in the domains of attention, verbal learning, verbal memory and executive functioning. Improvements in negative symptoms, quality of life and some aspects of everyday functioning were also observed. Participants in the treatment condition reported increased use of cognitive strategies, as well as general satisfaction with the intervention. Overall, this brief, low-tech, low-cost and portable cognitive training intervention seems to help individuals effectively incorporate practical cognitive strategies and habits in their daily lives.

Schizophrenia is often characterized by an individual's positive and negative symptoms. People suffering from this illness, however, commonly have cognitive impairments that can interfere with thinking and behavior [1, 2]. These deficits occur in the broad areas of attention, processing speed, working memory, learning, memory and executive function [3]. Cognition is related to functional skills such as vocational achievement, social competency and independent living [4–8]. Prior research has demonstrated that impairment on neuropsychological measures is directly related to functional outcome, as measured by functional skills assessment and self-report or collateral report of real-world functioning [8–10]. Just as positive and negative

The first 2 authors contributed equally to this chapter.

symptoms can affect an individual's ability to interact with the world, cognitive deficits can be debilitating and are deserving of targeted intervention. Amelioration of cognitive dysfunction, then, is an essential goal of treatment and rehabilitation for those with schizophrenia. Antipsychotic medications address mainly the positive symptoms of schizophrenia but have had little or no success in improving cognitive deficits [11]. Therefore, psychosocial interventions such as cognitive training (CT) are the current mainstay of cognitive treatment [12–14].

CT for individuals with schizophrenia follows earlier work in the traumatic brain injury field. Neurorehabilitation efforts began during World War I, when programs were designed to help returning soldiers compensate for their deficits with psychological and occupational interventions [15]. The field of experimental psychopathology added to the development of CT, revealing that reducing attentional demands or increasing rewards improved the performance of individuals with schizophrenia on various laboratory tasks [16–18]. Furthermore, cognition has been shown to be a modifiable target for treatment, adding to the growing body of literature that supports cognitive remediation to improve neuropsychological performance and ultimately community functioning [12, 19].

Theoretically, CT approaches fall into 1 of 3 categories: environmental modification, restoration and compensation. Environmental modification interventions attempt to reduce the cognitive demands in an individual's environment to optimize functioning. The types of environmental manipulation include using electronic or paper reminders in the home, clothing organization and planning, and provision of pillboxes, alarm clocks and the like [20]. Environmental approaches are generally therapist driven, with the therapist helping clients modify their surroundings to simplify daily activities. Although environmental approaches are generally effective due to personally relevant, easily implemented changes to a person's surroundings, the high degree of therapist involvement may be expensive, and assistance may be needed over a long period of time. Furthermore, the gains may not generalize to other environments outside the home. Restorative approaches, which rely on drills and practice of various tasks, aim to eliminate cognitive impairments by repairing underlying brain functioning. Restorative methods have been shown to normalize performance on certain neuropsychological tests and even brain activation as measured by functional neuroimaging, but evidence of generalization of treatment gains to daily functioning has been less compelling [21–23]. Compensatory approaches aim to help individuals 'work around' cognitive deficits by employing internal and external cognitive strategies, with the hope that the strategies become habitual over time. The goal of compensatory CT is to have clients initiate and carry out appropriate strategies in a variety of real-world settings; however, clients must self-initiate strategy use, which may not always happen. Within these 3 types of approaches, interventions may be group or individual, computer-assisted or not, stand-alone treatments or treatments embedded in psychosocial rehabilitation programs, and may focus on just 1 (e.g. attention) or many cognitive domains.

Our CT Intervention

Our CT approach combines compensatory strategy training with client-driven environmental modifications, with the hope that the intervention can be brief, low-tech, low-cost, portable, practical and generalizable to a wide variety of real-world situations. The goal of our intervention is to help clients develop strategies to form long-term habits that are meaningful in the real world. Habit learning may have several advantages: it is more similar to procedural learning than declarative memory [24, 25], it is intact in people with schizophrenia [26, 27], and it is resistant to forgetting [24].

Our manualized intervention is designed as a stand-alone, group-based treatment, although an individual manual is also available and is being tested within a supported employment program. The treatment is administered by 1–2 facilitators to groups of 4–8 people over 12 two-hour weekly sessions. We call it 'cognitive training class' rather than a 'group' to emphasize the skill-based nature of the intervention and to reduce stigma associated with 'group treatment'. Although it is a relatively brief intervention, it provides enough time for clients to practice strategies and consolidate new cognitive habits. Strategies are practiced through interactive, game-like activities to maintain interest and increase motivation; clients are also encouraged to identify personal goals to enhance intrinsic motivation and foster sustained attendance [28]. For example, clients might identify cognitive skills needed for success in their goals to achieve an educational objective, return to work, live more independently or enhance their interpersonal relationships. We target 4 neuropsychological domains: prospective memory, attention and vigilance, learning and memory, and executive functioning. These domains were selected based on their importance for everyday functioning and their modifiability [2, 8, 29]. Each session is designed to review homework and previous strategies, then introduce and practice new compensatory strategies and help clients develop individualized plans to implement the strategies in their daily lives. Key strategies in each domain are discussed in the 4 sections below. Homework is assigned each week to promote strategy use outside of class and to troubleshoot any barriers that arise. The CT manual employs ideas and materials from various sources, including the Acquired Brain Injury program at Mesa College in San Diego (calendar training and to-do lists), the social skills training manual (conversational vigilance skills, 6-step problem-solving method) by Bellack et al. [30], Meichenbaum and Cameron's [31] work on self-talk for task vigilance, and Delahunty and Morice's [32] manual, also used by Wykes et al. [33] (categorization tasks).

Prospective Memory

The first 3 sessions focus on prospective memory (i.e. remembering to remember), with strategies centered on calendar use and to-do lists. Daily calendar use is introduced in the first session and is reinforced throughout the remainder of the 12-week intervention. Calendars are provided to all clients so that they are able to start using them immediately. A variety of calendar sizes and formats are offered to ensure that clients will be able to carry their calendars everywhere they go. They are encouraged to check their calendar every day at a specific time, as well as set up a planning session once a week to add new appointments and review the upcoming schedule. Calendar entries are reviewed regularly to monitor the amount of detail necessary (e.g. enter 'Dr. Smith, lithium SE' at 10 am instead of 'meet with Dr. Smith at 10 am and ask about lithium side effects'). Clients are also taught how to create to-do lists and how to incorporate them into their calendar (e.g. using sticky notes that can be moved from week to week). During the second session, prioritizing to-do list tasks is introduced and practiced by assigning high-, medium- and low-priority categories to (1) sample daily activities that are provided in the manual and (2) lists of activities the clients create for their own actual use. Another prospective memory technique introduced in the second session is the concept of linking tasks, where clients are taught how to remember to do a new activity by pairing it with an activity they already do automatically (e.g. taking medication right after brushing your teeth). This strategy is used to form the habit of daily calendar checking. The use of 'can't miss reminders' is introduced in the second and third sessions. Placing reminders in areas the client will be sure to see increases the probability of accomplishing the desired task. These reminders can be written on sticky notes and placed on something the client is sure to touch during the day, written on the client's hand or left as a voice message on an answering machine. 'Automatic places' also enhance prospective memory, helping clients adhere to the principle of 'a place for everything and everything in its place' (e.g. always keep keys on hook near front door; always keep wallet on bedside table).

Attention and Vigilance

The next 3 sessions target conversational and task vigilance to help clients maintain focus and improve attention. Conversational vigilance is discussed in terms of 4 'golden rules': (1) eliminate distractions in the environment, (2) look at the person who is speaking, (3) paraphrase what is said, and (4) ask questions and ask the person to slow down or repeat the information when necessary. Time is spent practicing each of these steps in class, with clients engaging in conversations and testing their own ability to pay attention to the conversation, as well as to understand and remember what is said to them. Task vigilance techniques incorporate some of the rules the clients learned in the conversation vigilance section: paraphrasing and asking questions as well as the use of 'self-talk'. Clients are encouraged to say the steps of the task out loud while doing it in order to stay on task and avoid forgetting the main steps. Clients practice the self-talk technique while performing complex motor sequences and while deciding if the steps of common tasks are in the correct order.

Learning and Memory

The 3 learning and memory sessions concentrate on improving encoding and retrieving information, with a special emphasis on remembering names. One of the primary encoding strategies is note-taking, and clients are given assistance in fine-tuning their note-taking skills. Clients are asked to write down the essential parts of various directions or conversations that they may encounter in everyday life (e.g. instructions from physicians). The length and detail of their notes are reviewed to determine whether they need to write down more information or if they can reduce the amount of notes written. Other encoding techniques introduced in this section are paraphrasing, association of novel information with previously learned information, chunking, categorizing, acronyms, rhymes and overlearning. In addition, clients are asked to choose which techniques would be best to remember telephone numbers, names, dates, directions and other verbal information; they learn that there are multiple strategies for encoding all types of information and that note-taking is almost always a good option. The last encoding strategy introduced in this section is visual imagery; clients are taught to learn new names by using a visual image to help make that name more memorable, e.g. 'Dr. Burns has dark, stubbly hair, as if there had been a big brush fire (burn) on top of his head'. Retrieval strategies include relaxation, mental retracing, alphabetic searching and recreating the context in which the memory was encoded.

Executive Functioning

The remaining sessions target executive functioning, with a 6-step problem-solving method and detailed, personalized coaching on brainstorming. Clients practice brainstorming by generating 15–20 solutions to sample situations (e.g. all the materials needed for a child's birthday party; all the ways to get a cat out of a tree), then practice brainstorming solutions to self-identified problems (e.g. all the ways to look for a job; all the ways to learn the local bus routes; all the ways to save money). Generally, brainstorming and problem-solving examples begin with generic, less emotionally-laden topics and move to more personally relevant, real-world problems. Once the clients feel comfortable with brainstorming, they are asked to use the 6-step problem-solving method to find solutions to problems they have encountered. This method includes the following steps: (1) defining the problem, (2) brainstorming solutions, (3) evaluating the solutions on cost, ease of implementation and likelihood of success, (4) selecting a solution to try, (5) trying the solution, and (6) evaluating the solution. Clients are asked to identify at least 1 problem they would like to solve, and over the course of the next few sessions, class work as well as homework progresses through the 6-step problem-solving method (e.g. 'How can I increase my income?' 'How can I find a new place to live?'). Cognitive flexibility is also highlighted; clients are encouraged to monitor progress and change behavior accordingly through games like 20 questions and sorting decks of playing cards, and then plan how to apply these skills in their own lives. Other methods include strategy verbalization (i.e. using self-talk while solving problems), hypothesis testing (looking for confirming and disconfirming evidence), and self-monitoring (set maintenance and set-shifting when strategies are working or not working). Stimuli such as sequenced pictures, visuospatial reasoning puzzles and playing cards are used to practice these skills, and plans for using the skills in everyday life are discussed.

How We Evaluate Our CT Intervention

Whereas some interventions have 'trained to the test', our stimuli and strategies do not employ the cognitive tests used as outcome measures in our research. We measure outcomes immediately following the intervention as well as 3 months after to evaluate whether initial gains are strengthened or attenuated over time. Finally, in addition to changes on neuropsychological tests, we assess differences in psychiatric symptom severity, functional capacity, self-reported functioning and quality of life.

A randomized controlled trial was designed to investigate the effectiveness of CT for outpatients with severe mental illness [34]. Participants were diagnosed as having a primary psychotic disorder, aged 21 years or older, English speaking, had no central nervous system compromise other than psychosis, and were not currently abusing drugs or alcohol. Following baseline evaluation, they were randomly assigned to CT plus standard pharmacotherapy (CT) or standard pharmacotherapy alone (SP); additional assessment occurred at 3 months (immediate posttreatment) and 6 months (follow-up). The CT groups were led by a combination of doctoral-level, masters-level and bachelors-level staff, with facilitators supervised by EWT. The evaluations included a comprehensive battery of neuropsychological, clinical and functional measures to examine changes in cognition, symptom severity, functional capacity, self-reported everyday functioning and quality of life (table 1). Participants also completed a standardized self-report questionnaire of cognitive problems they encounter and strategies used to manage such difficulties (table 1).

Results of CT

The results from 38 participants who were included in the analyses are shown in tables 2 and 3. Participants assigned to the CT group attended 81% of the CT sessions. Effect size analyses [35] comparing 0- to 3-month and 0- to 6-month change scores in the CT and SP groups revealed medium to large positive effects of CT on the domains of attention, verbal learning, verbal memory and executive functioning. Certain aspects of everyday functioning (e.g. communication, household chores) were also positively affected by CT. CT had no influence on positive symptoms of psychosis,

Table 1. Domains and measures

Neuropsychological	
Prospective memory	Memory for Intentions Screening Test total score [Raskin, unpublished]
Attention/vigilance	Wechsler Adult Intelligence Scale Digit Span forward score [36]
Verbal learning	Hopkins Verbal Learning Test total recall [37]
Verbal memory	Hopkins Verbal Learning Test percent retained
Executive functioning	Wisconsin Card Sorting Test total correct [38]
Processing speed	Wechsler Adult Intelligence Scale Digit Symbol total correct
Working memory	Wechsler Adult Intelligence Scale Letter Number Sequencing total correct
Language	Animals, Fruits, Vegetables total correct [39]
Visual learning	Brief Visuospatial Memory Test total recall [40]
Visual memory	Brief Visuospatial Memory Test percent retained
Functional capacity	UCSD Performance-Based Skills Assessment [9]
Symptom severity	Positive and Negative Syndrome Scale [41]
Quality of life	Quality of Life Interview global satisfaction [42]
Cognitive strategy use	Cognitive Problems and Strategies Assessment [Twamley, unpublished]

but it did demonstrate large effects on negative symptoms at immediate posttreatment, as well as medium to large effects on subjective quality of life. In addition, CT participants reported increased cognitive strategy use following the intervention; effect sizes greater than 0.5 are summarized in table 4. Many of those influences were somewhat attenuated at follow-up; however, several effects were stronger at follow-up than at immediate posttreatment. This finding suggests that some initial gains may need reinforcement to be maintained, and some may be consolidated over time. The following participant quotes highlight the utility of CT in developing new cognitive strategies:

'My calendar helps me to mark off my morning pills – I can check to see that I took them.'

'[The calendar] gives me peace of mind. I make notes to myself about ordering prescriptions and household duties.'

'I went from not checking my sugars daily (maybe every other day or I would skip a few days) to checking every day or twice a day. I write my sugar levels down in my calendar' (from an individual with type II diabetes).

'Paraphrasing makes my conversations more interesting. Normally I would just say, "Is that right?", but now I'm a more active participant.'

Table 2. Effect sizes for objective measures: neuropsychological and functional capacity assessments

	Cohen's d	
	3 months	6 months
Targeted cognitive domains		
Prospective memory	0.22	0.47
Attention/vigilance	0.49	1.00
Verbal learning	0.38	0.67
Verbal memory	0.61	0.04
Executive functioning	0.47	0.79
Nontargeted cognitive domains		
Processing speed	−0.16	−0.41
Working memory	−0.16	−0.31
Language	0.15	−0.01
Visual learning	−0.86	−0.23
Visual memory	0.97	0.25
Functional capacity		
UPSA household chores	0.62	0.94
UPSA communication	0.48	0.57
UPSA finance	0.03	−0.04
UPSA transportation	0.09	0.21
UPSA planning recreational activities	−0.18	−0.18
UPSA total score	0.67	0.89

Cohen's d effect sizes compare mean CT change scores to mean SP change scores at 3 and 6 months. Positive effect sizes indicate improvement. UPSA = UCSD Performance-Based Skills Assessment.

'I love the overlearning strategy to remember names. I made flashcards for each new person I met at my AA meetings. On the back of the card, I'll write down their phone number and personal details… I'm having a social life outside of my addiction for the first time in two and a half years.'

'Self-talk is a learning tool. It's not like talking back to voices. If you do it for instructions or a task, it's normal.'

The results thus far from this compensatory CT intervention are encouraging. CT has been feasible to deliver and has been well received by participants; CT completers rated the intervention highly in terms of overall satisfaction (8.8 on a 1–10 scale), quality of instruction (9.5), likelihood of recommending the class to others (9.0) and feeling personally helped by the class as a whole (8.4). The ratings within the 4 modules were also positive: 8.8 for prospective memory and executive functioning, 8.6 for attention and vigilance, and 8.1 for learning and memory. CT has also proven to be

Table 3. Effect sizes for subjective measures: symptom severity, quality of life and cognitive strategy use

	Cohen's d	
	3 months	6 months
Symptoms		
PANSS positive symptoms	−0.04	0.12
PANSS negative symptoms	0.93	0.17
Quality of Life		
Quality of Life Interview global satisfaction	0.52	0.84
Cognitive problems and strategies assessment		
Mean of all cognitive strategies	1.27	1.06
Calendar use	1.59	1.19
Making lists	1.01	0.49
Writing things down	0.71	0.48
Mental imagery	0.69	0.55
Categorization	0.50	0.32
Overlearning	0.94	0.31
Paraphrasing	0.52	0.15
Making eye contact	0.97	0.85
Asking questions	1.06	0.76
Maintaining a daily schedule	1.14	0.43
Automatic places	0.87	0.87
Hypothesis testing	0.59	0.35
Set switching	0.65	0.90
Brainstorming solutions	0.42	0.62
Using a problem-solving method	0.33	0.50
Self-monitoring	0.28	0.62

Cohen's d effect sizes compare mean CT change scores to mean SP change scores at 3 and 6 months. Positive effect sizes indicate improvement. PANSS = Positive and Negative Syndrome Scale.

low cost, low tech and portable. The manualized nature of the intervention has made CT easy to administer without extensive formal training.

Recent literature suggests that CT or cognitive remediation is more effective as part of other psychosocial rehabilitation programs, like supported employment [12]; we are now evaluating a combined CT and supported employment intervention. Whether CT is used as a stand-alone intervention or as a part of other rehabilitative services, the hope is that cognitive strategies develop into long-term habits that generalize beyond the classroom and ultimately enhance independent living and community integration of individuals with severe mental illness.

References

1 Twamley EW, Dolder CR, Corey-Bloom J, Jeste DV: Neuropsychiatric aspects of schizophrenia. Neuropsychiatry 2003:776.

2 Green MF, Nuechterlein KH: Should schizophrenia be treated as a neurocognitive disorder? Schizophr Bull 1999;25:309.

3 Heinrichs RW, Zakzanis KK: Neurocognitive deficit in schizophrenia: a quantitative review of the evidence. Neuropsychology 1998;12:426–445.

4 McGurk SR, Mueser KT: Cognitive functioning, symptoms, and work in supported employment: a review and heuristic model. Schizophr Res 2004;70: 147–173.

5 Palmer BW, Heaton RK, Gladsjo JA, Evans JD, Patterson TL, Golshan S, Jeste DV: Heterogeneity in functional status among older outpatients with schizophrenia: employment history, living situation, and driving. Schizophr Res 2002;55:205–215.

6 Pinkham AE, Penn DL: Neurocognitive and social cognitive predictors of interpersonal skill in schizophrenia. Psychiatry Res 2006;143:167–178.

7 Brekke JS, Hoe M, Long J, Green MF: How neurocognition and social cognition influence functional change during community-based psychosocial rehabilitation for individuals with schizophrenia. Schizophr Bull 2007;33:1247–1256.

8 Twamley EW, Doshi RR, Nayak GV, Palmer BW, Golshan S, Heaton RK, Patterson TL, Jeste DV: Generalized cognitive impairments, ability to perform everyday tasks, and level of independence in community living situations of older patients with psychosis. Am J Psychiatry 2002;159:2013–2020.

9 Patterson TL, Goldman S, McKibbin CL, Hughs T, Jeste DV: UCSD performance-based skills assessment: development of a new measure of everyday functioning for severely mentally ill adults. Schizophr Bull 2001;27:235.

10 Bowie CR, Twamley EW, Anderson H, Halpern B, Patterson TL, Harvey PD: Self-assessment of functional status in schizophrenia. J Psychiatr Res 2007; 41:1012–1018.

11 Goldberg TE, Goldman RS, Burdick KE, Malhotra AK, Lencz T, Patel RC, Woerner MG, Schooler NR, Kane JM, Robinson DG: Cognitive improvement after treatment with second-generation antipsychotic medications in first-episode schizophrenia: is it a practice effect? Arch Gen Psychiatry 2007;64: 1115.

12 McGurk SR, Twamley EW, Sitzer DI, McHugo GJ, Mueser KT: A meta-analysis of cognitive remediation in schizophrenia. Am J Psychiatry 2007;164: 1791–1802.

13 Roder V, Mueller DR, Mueser KT, Brenner HD: Integrated psychological therapy (IPT) for schizophrenia: is it effective? Schizophr Bull 2006;32:S81.

14 Kurtz MM: Neurocognitive rehabilitation for schizophrenia. Curr Psychiatry Rep 2003;5:303–310.

15 Goldstein K: Aftereffects of Brain Injuries in War: Their Evaluation and Treatment; the Application of Psychologic Methods in the Clinic. New York, Grune & Stratton, 1942.

16 Cromwell RL: Assessment of schizophrenia. Annu Rev Psychol 1975;26:593–619.

17 Cromwell RL, Spaulding W: How schizophrenics handle information. Phenomenol Treat Schizophr 1978:127–162.

18 Spaulding WD, Storms L, Goodrich V, Sullivan M: Applications of experimental psychopathology in psychiatric rehabilitation. Schizophr Bull 1986;12: 560.

19 Twamley EW, Jeste DV, Bellack AS: A review of cognitive training in schizophrenia. Schizophr Bull 2003;29:359–382.

20 Velligan DI, Prihoda TJ, Ritch JL, Maples N, Bow-Thomas CC, Dassori A: A randomized single-blind pilot study of compensatory strategies in schizophrenia outpatients. Schizophr Bull 2002;28:283.

21 Fiszdon JM, Bryson GJ, Wexler BE, Bell MD: Durability of cognitive remediation training in schizophrenia: performance on two memory tasks at 6-month and 12-month follow-up. Psychiatry Res 2004;125:1–7.

22 Wexler BE, Anderson M, Fulbright RK, Gore JC: Preliminary evidence of improved verbal working memory performance and normalization of task-related frontal lobe activation in schizophrenia following cognitive exercises. Am J Psychiatry 2000: 1694–1697.

23 Fisher M, Holland C, Subramaniam K, Vinogradov S: Neuroplasticity-based cognitive training in schizophrenia: an interim report on the effects 6 months later. Schizophr Bull, in press (epub ahead of print).

24 Bayley PJ, Frascino JC, Squire LR: Robust habit learning in the absence of awareness and independent of the medial temporal lobe. Nature 2005;436: 550–553.

25 Knowlton BJ, Mangels JA, Squire LR: A neostriatal habit learning system in humans. Science 1996;273: 1399.

26 Clare L, McKenna PJ, Mortimer AM, Baddeley AD: Memory in schizophrenia: what is impaired and what is preserved? Neuropsychologia 1993;31:1225.

27 Keri S, Juhasz A, Rimanoczy A, Szekeres G, Kelemen O, Cimmer C, Szendi I, Benedek G, Janka Z: Habit learning and the genetics of the dopamine D3 receptor: evidence from patients with schizophrenia and healthy controls. Behav Neurosci 2005;119:687–693.

28 Choi J, Medalia A: Factors associated with a positive response to cognitive remediation in a community psychiatric sample. Psychiatr Serv 2005;56:602.

29 Green MF: What are the functional consequences of neurocognitive deficits in schizophrenia? Am J Psychiatry 1996:321–330.

30 Bellack AS, Mueser KT, Gingerich S, Agresta J: Social Skills Training for Schizophrenia. New York, Guilford Press, 1997.

31 Meichenbaum D, Cameron R: Training schizophrenics to talk to themselves: a means of developing attentional controls. Behavr Ther 1973;4:515–534.

32 Delahunty A, Morice R: A Training Programme for the Remediation of Cognitive Deficits in Schizophrenia. Albury, Department of Health, 1993.

33 Wykes T, Reeder C, Corner J, Williams C, Everitt B: The effects of neurocognitive remediation on executive processing in patients with schizophrenia. Schizophr Bull 1999;25:291.

34 Twamley EW, Savla GN, Zurhellen CH, Heaton RK, Jeste DV: Development and pilot testing of a novel compensatory cognitive training intervention for people with psychosis. Am J Psychiatr Rehabil 2008;11:144–163.

35 Cohen J: Statistical Power Analysis for the Behavioral Sciences. Hillsdale, Lawrence Erlbaum Associates, 1988.

36 Wechsler D: Wechsler Adult Intelligence Scale – Third Edition (WAIS-III). San Antonio, Psychological Corporation, 1997.

37 Benedict RHB, Schretlen D, Groninger L, Brandt J: Hopkins Verbal Learning Test – revised: normative data and analysis of inter-form and test-retest reliability. Clin Neuropsychol 1998;12:43–55.

38 Kongs SK, Thompson LL, Iverson GL, Heaton RK: Wisconsin Card Sorting Test-64 Card Version (WCST-64). Odessa, Psychological Assessment Resources, 2000.

39 Benton AL, Hamsher K: Multilingual Aphasia Examination. Iowa City, AJA Associates, 1989.

40 Benedict RHB: Brief Visual-Spatial Memory Test – Revised. Professional Manual. Odessa, Psychological Assessment Resources, 1997.

41 Kay SR, Opler LA, Fiszbein A: Positive and Negative Syndrome Scale (PANSS) Rating Manual. San Rafael, Social and Behavioral Sciences Documents, 1987.

42 Lehman AF: A quality of life interview for the chronically mentally ill. Eval Program Plann 1988;11:51–62.

Elizabeth W. Twamley, PhD
University of California, San Diego
140 Arbor Drive (0851)
San Diego, CA 92103 (USA)
Tel. +1 619 497 6684, Fax +1 619 497 6686, E-Mail etwamley@ucsd.edu

Roder V, Medalia A (eds): Neurocognition and Social Cognition in Schizophrenia Patients. Basic Concepts and Treatment. Key Issues Ment Health. Basel, Karger, 2010, vol 177, pp 61–78

4

Treatment Approaches with a Special Focus on Social Cognition: Overview and Empirical Results

Wolfgang Wölwer[a] · Dennis R. Combs[b] · Nicole Frommann[a] · David L. Penn[c]

[a]Department of Psychiatry and Psychotherapy, Heinrich Heine University Düsseldorf, Rhineland State Clinics Düsseldorf, Düsseldorf, Germany; [b]Department of Psychology and Counseling, University of Texas at Tyler, Tyler, Tex., and [c]Department of Psychology, University of North Carolina at Chapel Hill, Chapel Hill, N.C., USA

Abstract

Impairments in social cognition have become an increasingly important area to target for intervention studies, mainly because (a) such impairments are closely associated with poor social and community functioning and (b) are stable across the course of schizophrenia despite clinically effective antipsychotic drug and psychosocial treatment. During the past years a number of special treatment programs have been designed to directly address impairments in social cognition, usually considering them to be 'deficits' rather than 'biases'. Such programs apply cognitive-remediation style intervention techniques to the processing of social information and can be characterized as either more 'targeted' or more 'broad-based'. The most targeted intervention approaches seek to improve a single aspect of social cognition, while more broad-based strategies have a number of social cognitive targets, and/or also address basic cognitive processes like attention and memory, and/or additionally include social behavioral skill training. Although social cognitive remediation is still in an infant stage of development, the initial efficacy results are encouraging, showing that improvements in social cognition can be obtained by a variety of specific intervention approaches. In contrast, standard neurocognitive training alone seems neither necessary nor sufficient to improve social cognitive processes.

Social Cognition in Schizophrenia

Social cognition can be generally defined as the 'mental operations underlying social interactions, which include the human ability and capacity to perceive the intentions and dispositions of others' [1–3]. Adolphs [4] further defined social cognition as 'the ability to construct representations of the relation between oneself and others and to use those representations flexibly to guide social behavior' (p. 231). These definitions

Table 1. Domains of social cognition

	Description	Representative measures
Theory of Mind	Ability to represent the mental states of others or make inferences about others' intentions; this includes understanding hints, false beliefs, intentions, irony, metaphor and faux pas	Hinting Task Brüne Cartoons Test of Awareness of Social Inference
Attributional style	Assigning causality to positive and negative events	Internal, Personal and Situational Attributions Questionnaire Ambiguous Intentions Hostility Questionnaire
Emotion perception	Perception or scanning of social details and scenes Identification or discrimination of emotional expressions; emotional expressions usually reflect both positive (happy and surprise) and negative emotional states (anger, fear, sadness, ashamed, disgust)	Face Emotion Identification Test Bell-Lysaker Emotion Recognition Test Ekman Faces
Social perception	Perception or scanning of social details/cues and use of context	Profile of Nonverbal Sensitivity Social Perception Scale

share the idea that social cognition is a set of cognitive processes that are related and applied to the recognition, understanding and accurate processing of social information and interactions [1].

In the area of schizophrenia, there are 4 primary areas that define social cognition [5, 6]. They include: (1) emotion perception, (2) social perception, (3) theory of mind (ToM) and (4) attributional style. Table 1 presents definitions and representative measures of each area. There is now comprehensive evidence that patients suffering from schizophrenia are impaired in each of these social cognitive domains [e.g. 2, 7]. However, it is still under discussion whether these impairments have to be conceptualized in a quantitative manner as 'deficits' or qualitatively as 'biases'. Deficit models originated from neuropsychological research and interpret social cognitive impairments in the sense of inabilities or restriction of abilities, whereas bias models originated from social psychological research and suggest such impairments to be errors in judgment due to some kind of distorted usage of (actually existing) abilities. For example, the latter approaches assume that schizophrenia patients – in particular those with delusions – misinterpret social information because they excessively attend to threatening information, often jump to conclusions on the basis of insufficient information and attribute negative events preferably to external personal causes [8]. However, considerable heterogeneity across patients suffering from schizophrenia exists, and deficits as well as biases may exist and contribute to maladaptive social functioning.

Wölwer · Combs · Frommann · Penn

Social cognition has become an increasingly important area to target for intervention studies for a number of reasons. First, it appears to be an independent construct that is different from neurocognition [9] and psychotic symptoms [10] and that is controlled by a special 'social cognitive neural circuit'. This neural network includes the amygdala, fusiform gyrus, superior temporal sulcus and prefrontal cortices [7]. Secondly, impairments in social cognition are stable across the course of schizophrenia despite clinically effective antipsychotic drug and psychosocial treatment [11, 12]. Thirdly and most importantly, social cognition has a robust association with social and community functioning [13]. In fact, there are now a large number of studies that demonstrate that social cognition is a direct predictor [14–17], mediator [18, 19] or moderator [20] of social and community functioning. In addition, some investigations have shown that social cognition has a stronger relationship with functional outcome than neurocognition [21–23].

Special Treatment Approaches for Social Cognition

Depending on whether poorer social cognitive performance in schizophrenia is conceptualized as a cognitive 'deficit' or as a cognitive 'bias', either remediation or debiasing intervention approaches need to be employed. However, bias models and thus debiasing strategies have not exerted very much influence on the development of social cognitive treatment yet. Cognitive behavioral therapy for positive symptoms [e.g. 24] have adopted such debiasing strategies, but empirical evaluations most often used positive symptoms as primary outcome rather than social cognitive performance [25, 26]. Only recently did debiasing approaches addressing social cognitive processes as primary target and primary outcome come into the focus of research. For example the Meta-Cognitive Training [27], an 8-session group intervention for 3–10 patients each, tries to modify cognitive biases by making patients aware of these biases and their association with delusions, by demonstrating the negative consequences of cognitive biases to the patients and by instructing them to critically reflect and change their behavior so far. As its evaluation is still ongoing, no conclusions about the efficacy of such a debiasing approach can be drawn yet.

Most other treatment programs designed to directly address impairments in social cognition implicitly or explicitly consider the impairments to be 'deficits'. These approaches apply cognitive-remediation style intervention techniques to the processing of social information and can be characterized as either more 'targeted' or more 'broad-based'. The most targeted intervention approaches seek to improve a single aspect of social cognition (e.g. emotion perception or ToM), while more broad-based ones have a number of targets for improvement either within the social cognitive domain (e.g. emotion perception and ToM), beyond the borders of social cognition by explicitly also addressing neurocognition or even beyond the borders of cognitive processes by including behavioral processes, in particular social behavioral skills.

Such broader approaches typically also involve a variety of psychosocial intervention methods [13]. Due to the multiple criteria regarding targets and intervention methods potentially characterizing more broad-based approaches, the differentiation between broad-based and targeted should be taken as end points of a continuum rather than as a strict categorical distinction.

In the following, broad-based interventions will be defined as treatments that: (1) are comprised of a number of different interventions, such as packaging neurocognitive remediation methods with social cognitive or social skill training, and/or (2) are directed towards improving multiple areas of social cognition. Only intervention programs explicitly targeting social cognitive processes will be included – treatment approaches intending to primarily improve social behavioral skills (e.g. Social Skill Training) probably also affect underlying social cognitive processes indeed, but the effects of such an implicit training have rarely been investigated with regard to cognitive outcomes.

Targeted Intervention Approaches

Overview and Empirical Results

The pioneering approaches in the development of explicit remediation strategies for social cognitive impairments were interventions targeting only 1 social cognitive domain. These approaches for the first time proved that it is possible to modify social cognitive functions by training.

One of the first attempts of targeted remediation in social cognition concerned ToM function [28, 29] and showed that the technique of verbalization helps improve performance in the character intention task – a novel nonverbal ToM task. Subsequent intervention approaches mainly focused on affect recognition, which is suggested to be a basic building block of social cognition and communication [7]. The first intervention study concerning affect recognition was conducted by Penn and Combs [30]. They demonstrated in 4 groups of schizophrenia inpatients (in total 40 subjects) that monetary reinforcement, facial feedback and a combination of reinforcement and facial feedback, but not repeated practice, can improve affect recognition performance already within a single training session. However, the gains for each intervention were poorly maintained at a follow-up 1 week after the training session. In a similar randomized controlled trial comprising 60 schizophrenia inpatients, Combs et al. [31] showed that attentional shaping significantly improves facial affect recognition even beyond contingent monetary reinforcement and repeated practice. Based on evidence for an association between affect recognition and attention [e.g. 11] and other evidence pointing to restricted visual scan paths often neglecting the essential areas of the face [e.g. 32, 33], the attentional shaping training tried to focus on the eye and mouth areas of the face by presenting a large cross in the center of the emotional face as a prompt. Though the training comprised just 1 session as in its predecessor study, the gain proved to be stable at a 1 week follow-up. However, as no healthy control group was investigated, the clinical significance remains unclear, i.e. whether posttreatment performance reached healthy norm levels or continued to be impaired.

Another single-session training used the computer-based Microexpression Training Tool (METT) [34]. Microexpressions are rapid 15-millisecond 'flashes' of facial affect beginning and ending with a neutral face. The training started with slow-motion video sequences of commonly confused emotions in order to explain important distinctions between the basic facial affect expressions. Thereafter, the participants had to label 28 trials of microexpressions with feedback provided. Incorrect trials led to a repetition of the trial or a still picture display of the emotion in order to correct the response. The patients trained with the METT showed a significant improvement in performance with posttreatment scores almost reaching the pretreatment performance level of healthy controls [34]. These positive effects could be replicated in a later study comparing METT training with a repeated exposure condition [35]. This study also provided evidence that improvements in facial affect recognition were associated with changes in visual scanning towards more attending to the feature areas of the face. However, in contrast to the more enduring influence of METT regarding recognition performance, effects regarding visual scanning behavior attenuated to a trend at a 1-week follow-up.

Silver et al. [36] adapted a computerized emotion training program, the Emotional Trainer, originally developed for teaching autistic children. The authors examined the effects of three 15-min sessions, spaced 2–3 days apart in 20 stable chronic schizophrenia patients and reported postintervention affect recognition to be better than at baseline. However, as they used an uncontrolled pre-post design, the informative value of this study is limited.

A more extended training program primarily targeting affect recognition has been developed by Frommann et al. [37] and Wölwer et al. [38]. Details of this manualized 12-session Training of Affect Recognition (TAR) shall be provided in the subsequent section. The TAR was first evaluated in a randomized controlled trial in 77 postacute patients with schizophrenia [38]. A pre-post control group design was used comprising both an active control group treated with a Cognitive Remediation Training (CRT) aiming at improvement of basic neurocognitive functioning and a 'passive' control group treated as usual without any cognitive training. Facial affect recognition, face recognition and basic cognitive functioning were assessed as outcome measures. Analyses revealed specific training effects in the form of a double dissociation: the TAR improved facial affect recognition but had no effects on memory, attention and executive functioning, whereas patients under CRT and those without training did not show improvements in affect recognition. However, patients under CRT improved in verbal learning and memory. Positive effects of the TAR on affect recognition were replicated in 2 successive studies comparing the TAR either against

CRT or against a waiting group [39]. These studies also obtained evidence that the gains maintain for at least 6–8 weeks after the end of training and that improvements also occur in prosodic affect recognition and – to a lesser extent – in ToM. However, an immediate impact on social interaction as assessed by a role play test could not be found. According to these results, improvements in disturbed facial affect recognition in schizophrenia patients are not obtainable with a traditional cognitive remediation program like CRT but need a functional specific training of social cognition.

The Example of the TAR

The TAR primarily aims to improve impairments in decoding facial affect in patients suffering from schizophrenia. The training program comprises both restitution and compensation methods, i.e. beyond repeated practice it also tries to establish alternative strategies of information processing known to be essential both for the efficacy of remediation approaches and for the generalization of effects [40]. Core principles applied in TAR are
- errorless learning [41], i.e. the avoidance of the occurrence of errors during the training phase,
- overlearning, i.e. frequent repetition of facial features prototypical of basic emotions,
- immediate (verbal) positive feedback and
- feature abstraction, i.e. abstraction from individual to prototypical expressions.

These core principles are combined with alternative, compensatory cognitive strategies such as verbalization, self-instruction and the generation of associations using situational clues as well as context information. The TAR is a manualized program of 12 structured sessions, applied twice weekly for about 1 h per training session to pairs of patients at a time. About half of the tasks are computer based, while the others are presented as desk work. A playful character of the computer-based tasks is intended to improve motivation and compliance. To boost generalization of training content into everyday life, homework is given between each session, and every session starts with reviewing the homework. After 4 sessions each, patients have to perform short tests in order to monitor learning progress.

The sessions are led by a therapist who supports and guides the patients through the tasks by coaching methods and by applying the training principles mentioned above. Since most tasks are executed by the patients in teamwork, the therapist has to manage performance and interaction of the pair in order to maximize profit for both, also paying regard to actual psychopathological symptoms which may restrict the training. Thus effective application of such training needs clinical as well as psychotherapeutic (especially cognitive behavior) expertise.

The TAR consists of 3 blocks of 4 sessions each, differing in primary content. Blocks 2 and 3 build on the preceding block. Table 2 summarizes contents and methods per

Table 2. TAR Sessions and Training Methods

	Session focus	Primary training methods
Sessions 1–4	Successive learning of basic emotions and their prototypical units of facial expression	Feature abstraction Discrimination learning Labeling Self-instructions
Sessions 5–8	Increase of speed and load of processing Promotion of holistic and nonverbal processing Decoding of expressions with varying and with low intensity	Reduction of presentation time Usage of degraded stimuli Focus on overall impression Matching Identification of most prominent features
Sessions 9–12	Decoding of ambiguous and nonprototypical facial expressions Interpretation of expressive behavior in social interaction	Reasoning based on feature abstraction Situative anchors Generation of associations between emotions, cognitions and situative context Consideration of other nonverbal expression (gestures, body posture)
General	Overlearning of basic emotions and their prototypical facial units	Repetitive practice Errorless learning Immediate positive feedback Verbalization

block, however, methods applied in more than 1 block are only mentioned in the block of main usage.

During the first 4 sessions the primary focus is to discriminate the prototypical facial expressions of basic emotions. The features of these emotions are presented by their typical mimic signs (action units) as described in the Facial Acting Coding System [42]and are verbalized using colloquial speech. The act of breaking down facial expressions into its details is intended to enhance the processing depth and promote the use of verbal prompts as an alternative decoding strategy to the usual holistic decoding.

Teaching basic emotions within the first TAR block starts with desk work contrasting each 2 of the basic emotions. Computer tasks presenting pictures of only the upper or lower parts of faces (e.g. only the mouth of a sad face or only the eyes of a surprised face) support this stage of training. Using only parts of the face has the advantage of reducing distracting information and promoting focus on the distinct features. However, complete pictures of faces are also used during this first block. Each task becomes successively more complex and difficult by presenting more items simultaneously. The 2 participants have to decide together and to justify their decision in order to practice verbalization of the typical facial features of the basic emotions.

One of the aims of the second block (sessions 5–8) is to return to and practice holistic processing based on first impression. Participants are asked to verify their first impression by reasoning and to resort to the alternative strategies learned in the first block in case of uncertainty. Computer-aided tasks with reduced display time or with degraded information were designed to facilitate this stage of training. Also nonverbal processing is promoted by tasks requiring matching emotions rather than using a labeling approach. A further aim of this block is to learn to decode different intensities of emotional expression, since affect expression in real life often does not occur with peak intensities like those displayed in the usual prototypical pictures but in rather low intensities. Pictures of facial affect which are morphed in varying proportions with neutral faces are used to obtain this aim (similarly to fig. 1 but using different persons).

The main objective of the third block (sessions 9–12) is the integration of affect recognition performance and the learned strategies into social interaction context as required in everyday life. So-called 'anchor tasks' referring to context information like situational background, accompanying nonverbal signs beyond facial expression, and associated cognitions are introduced. For example pictures of facial affect have to be matched to appropriate short descriptions of social situations and/or to the statement of thoughts possibly co-occurring during the emotion. Typical congruence between these information sources is explained and exercised in several tasks both at the desk and at the computer. Also nonprototypical, mixed emotions as well as ambiguous scenes are evaluated by referring to elements of basic emotions and by applying previously learned strategies.

Broad-Based Intervention Approaches

Overview and Empirical Results

One of the most prominent broad-based treatment approaches is the Integrated Psychological Therapy (IPT), which will be described in detail in a succession chapter (see [43] for a recent review of IPT). However, in terms of social cognition, only the social perception subprogram of IPT (program 2) is directed toward improving social and emotion recognition and emotional expression. Since researchers can select which of the 5 programs to administer, many studies have not included the social perception program and thus have focused more on cognitive change than social cognitive change [43]. More recent studies [44] have developed their own set of cognitive and social cognitive remediation activities or modified IPT methods [45] to produce change. In contrast to traditional IPT or cognitive remediation studies, a new class of purely social cognitive intervention has emerged. For example, Social Cognition and Interaction Training (SCIT) provides training in emotion perception, social problem solving, and generating accurate attributions for social situations and does not contain traditional neurocognitive exercises such as memory or attention training. Thus,

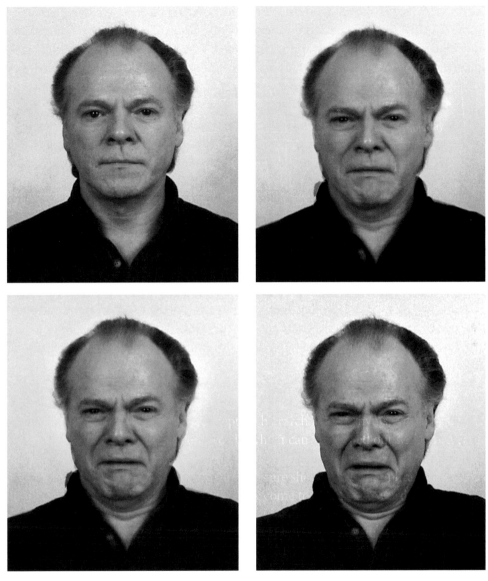

Fig. 1. Examples of emotion morph slides from SCIT (session 6). Note: participants are asked to identify each emotion and rate how confident they are in their guess on a scale of 1 to 10. Expressions increase in saliency from neutral to very intense.

at a conceptual level, such broad based treatments can be viewed as either top down (social cognitive processes or even metacognitive processes) or bottom up (neurocognitive processes) in terms of they foster change in social functioning.

There are a number of broad based studies and we will focus on those that have social cognitive aspects in the intervention methods. For a comprehensive review of the studies in this area, see Horan et al. [46].

Van der Gaag et al. [47] randomly assigned forty two participants to either a cognitive remediation intervention or a leisure skills group. The cognitive remediation intervention lasted 22 sessions and was delivered over a 3 month period of time. The intervention was comprised of four parts: (1) self-instructional training, (2) memory enhancement training, (3) inductive reasoning practice, and (4) compensatory strategy training. Training in social cognition and emotion perception occurred in the compensatory strategy training phase and lasted 6 sessions (sessions 17–22 for a total of 120 min). In those sessions, participants worked on emotion and social scene recognition, facial feature recognition, facial mimicry, and engaged in role-plays. Results showed that the cognitive remediation group had significantly higher scores on a task of emotion labeling and emotion matching as compared to the leisure skills group.

Hodel et al. [45] developed the Emotion Management Training (EMT) to improve emotion perception, social adjustment, and reduce the impact of stress on psychopathology. Twenty-two participants were assigned to 12 weeks of EMT (n = 11) or a problem solving group (n = 11). At post-treatment, the EMT group showed gains on emotion perception, social adjustment as measured by the NOSIE, and the BPRS to assess symptoms. At a 4 month follow-up, gains on the emotion perception test returned to baseline levels, but gains on social adjustment and psychopathology were maintained. At present, EMT has been effective in outpatient [48] and first-episode [49] samples as well.

Hogarty et al. [50] randomly assigned 121 persons with schizophrenia to either Cognitive Enhancement Therapy (CET) or a supportive therapy condition. Outcomes were measured at 12 and 24 months. CET was developed using concepts and methods from Ben-Yishay's rehabilitation work with traumatic brain injury (TBI) patients, IPT, and research on cognitive skills development. The main premise of CET is to move social cognition from a serial, effortful process to more of an automatic, gistful process. Social cognition training was provided in small groups that meet weekly in months 4 to 6 of CET (cognitive training was conducted first). In these groups, members discussed real-life social situations, practiced social skill exercises, conducted emotional expression activities, and discussed how context influences emotional reactions. At 12 months, participants in the CET condition showed improved cognition (neurocognition and processing speed composite scores) and social adjustment with a trend for improved social cognition ratings on a composite scale of 50 items rated by non-blinded clinicians. However, at 24 months, participants in CET showed significantly better social cognition ratings.

In a follow-up study by Eack et al. [51], thirty eight persons with early episode schizophrenia were randomly assigned to 12 months of CET or enhanced supportive therapy. Results showed that the CET group had greater scores on a performance based measure of emotional intelligence, the Mayer-Salvoy-Caruso Emotional Intelligence Test (MSCEIT, [52]), which is part of the MATRICS battery. CET participants improved in their ability to understand emotions, manage emotions, use emotions in decision making, and a trend was found for better perception of emotions.

More recent interventions are purely social cognitive in nature and are designed around activities to improve emotion perception, ToM, and attributional style. An example is the 'Training of Emotional Intelligence' (TEI, [53]) which will be described in detail in a subsequent chapter.

The 'Social Cognition Enhancement Training' (SCET, [54]) is a three level training system focusing on training in social cognitive abilities such as context appraisal and perspective-taking abilities. Each level consists of 12 sessions. The 36 sessions of one and a half hour are presented twice weekly about six months. Four-column cartoons are employed as major training material in social cognitive exercises in which participants are encouraged to perceive social cues in each piece of the cartoon, arrange the four pieces in order based on contextual information, and provide coherent explanations of the social situation depicted in the cartoon. In addition, SCET also tries to promote social problem solving strategies like discussing how to solve problems in a social situation similar to that depicted in the cartoon. The first evaluation of the SCET showed that a 6 month training improved contextual processing, but led to only small effects in social sequencing or emotion perception [54].

Social Cognition and Interaction Training (SCIT) is a further example of a broad-based social cognitive intervention. We will provide a detailed example of SCIT in the next section. Unlike, IPT or cognitive remediation studies, these social cognitive interventions are based on the assumption that social functioning can be improved directly by targeting social cognition. SCIT is a 20-week group-based intervention that has demonstrated efficacy in 2 small studies with inpatients [55, 56] and outpatients [57] with schizophrenia. A limitation of SCIT is that the 3 current studies are quasi-experimental in design and are not randomized controlled clinical trials (i.e. Penn and Combs are currently conducting a randomized controlled trial on SCIT funded by the National Institute of Mental Health). SCIT has shown some promise in improving ToM in adults with high-functioning autism as well [58].

Combs et al. [55] compared SCIT to a coping skills group in a sample of 28 forensic inpatients with schizophrenia. A total of 18 persons completed SCIT and 10 the coping skills group. Assignment was not random. At posttreatment, participants who completed SCIT showed robust improvements on emotion perception, ToM and less hostile attributions. In addition, there was better self-reported social functioning and less behavioral aggression. Unexpectedly, SCIT led to improvements on the Trail Making Test (measure of cognitive flexibility) even though there was no practice or training of this skill in the intervention. Persons in the coping skills group did not show gains on any of the measures. In a recent 6-month follow-up study on the SCIT group, it was found that scores did decrease from posttreatment to follow-up, but the gains were still higher than the pretest levels [59]. More importantly, there were no differences between SCIT participants and a matched nonclinical community sample. Roberts and Penn [57] examined SCIT in a sample of 31 outpatients with schizophrenia and found that persons who completed SCIT (n = 20) showed better scores on emotion perception and social skill ratings than those who received treatment as usual (n = 11). There were no changes in ToM or attributional style. The lack of more significant findings can be attributed to the use of outpatient samples who upon entry have higher levels of functioning than inpatients (possible ceiling effect).

At the University of California at Los Angeles, Horan et al. [60] randomly assigned 31 participants with schizophrenia to either a 12-session social cognitive intervention or a symptom management intervention. The 12-week social cognitive intervention consisted of two, 6-session phases. Phase 1 focused on emotion and social perception training and comprised repeated exercises in understanding and recognizing different emotional expressions, practice in facial mimicry, perception of nonverbal behaviors and understanding social norms. The activities involved the use of slide show presentations, as well as didactic and group discussion. Emotional expressions were presented in both still picture and video format to enhance the generalization of the training to real-world interactions. Phase 2 focused on attribution and ToM activities. The subjects of these sessions were paranoia, making good guesses about social situations, avoiding jumping to conclusions, how to check out your guesses and integrating information from all sources to understand interactions (e.g. use of the 5 W questions, who, what, when, where and why). This phase also contained work on the use of sarcasm and deception. Horan et al. [60] used methods and procedures from both SCIT and TAR to develop and refine the 12-week intervention. The results showed that at posttest, the scores on emotion perception significantly improved compared to the symptom management group. However, the scores on measures of attributional style, social perception and social inference were not higher. Changes in symptoms and neurocognition did not relate to the improvements in emotion perception. It is possible that the short duration of the treatment may not have been intensive enough to produce change in some of the more complex social cognitive abilities, and the authors are working on developing a 24-session intervention.

The Example of the SCIT

Social Cognition and Interaction Training (SCIT) is a comprehensive, 'stand-alone' manual-based intervention [61] that targets the 3 core social cognitive deficits in schizophrenia: emotion perception, ToM and attributional style [see 62]. SCIT is comprised of 3 phases and lasts 20–24 weeks (see table 3 for SCIT phases). SCIT is built around a 50-min group therapy session. The recommended group size is between 5 and 8 members with 2 group leaders and is appropriate for both in- and outpatients. SCIT involves the use of didactic instruction, videotape and computerized learning tools, and role play methods to improve social cognition. Weekly homework assignments are provided in the manual, and the group can involve 'practice partners' who work with the participant during the week. Each practice partner has information (handout is provided) about the session, its goals, what the person should have learned and specific activities to do together. The purpose of the practice partner is to

Table 3. SCIT sessions and activities

SCIT components	Session focus	Example of activity
Phase 1: emotions	*Emotion recognition*	
Sessions 1 and 2	Introduction	SCIT triangle; video examples
Session 3	Emotion and social situations	Practice scenarios
Session 4	Defining emotions	Emotion poster
Session 5	Guess Other's Emotions	Emotion trainer
Session 6	Updating emotion guesses	Emotion morph slides
Session 7	Suspicious feelings	Justified versus unjustified paranoia; video examples
Phase 2: figuring out situations	*ToMd and attributional style*	
Session 8	Jumping to conclusions	Video vignettes
Sessions 9 and 10	Thinking up other guesses	Discussion of 3 characters – My-Fault Mary, Blaming Bill and Easy Eddie
Sessions 11–13	Separate facts from guesses	Facts, guesses, emotions table for social situations
Sessions 14 and 15	Gather more evidence	Twenty-questions game
Phase 3: checking it out	*Emotion Recognition, ToM and Attributional Style*	
Sessions 16–20	Applying skills to real-life situations	Check it out process using facts, guesses and feelings Deciding what action to take Video vignettes

increase the generalization of SCIT and to provide more opportunities to practice the skills learned in the group.

Each SCIT session begins with a 10-min group check-in where members discuss how they are feeling (participants are asked 'are you feeling mostly good, mostly bad or neutral?'). The check-in provides examples for SCIT leaders to draw upon if needed and promotes awareness of emotional reactions (to help address possible alexithymia). After check-in, the leaders review the previous week's homework and then begin the material for the current session.

The primary goals of phase 1 (emotion training) are to provide information about emotions and their relationship to thoughts and situations, define the basic emotions, improve emotion perception skills with computerized facial expression training tools, and teach clients to distinguish between justified and unjustified suspiciousness.

Sessions 1–3 are built around the SCIT triangle, which is a concept adapted from cognitive therapy in which cognitions, behaviors and emotions are inter-related (e.g. multiple paths of causality). In session 4, the basic emotions of happiness, sadness, fear, anger, disgust and surprise are defined, and an emotions poster is created. The concept of paranoia as an emotion is added at this point (later the focus of session 7) due to the emotional reactions associated with paranoia in many SCIT participants. In session 5, we present participants with different facial displays of emotions (guessing others' emotions slide show) and ask them the following questions: (1) what makes him/her look that way?, or (2) what about him/her are you noticing? This information is added to the emotions poster to provide specific facial features or clues associated with each emotion. After examining facial features, the participants then select which emotion is being presented and provide a confidence level rating about their guess (0–100% sure), which is a type of metacognitive activity. In session 6, dynamic emotion morph slides are used, which shows how emotional expressions change from neutral to very intense (see fig. 1). At each step, clients are asked to make their best guess about the emotion and then rate their confidence on a scale of 1 to 10. The slides can be moved forward and backward to show subtle changes in emotions from neutral. Session 7 addresses paranoia and participants discuss different types of paranoia. For example, paranoia can be justified or unjustified, and determining intention is more difficult in ambiguous situations.

The primary goals of phase 2 (figuring out situations) are to teach clients about the potential pitfalls of jumping to conclusions, to improve cognitive flexibility in social situations, as well as to help them distinguish between personal and situational attributions, and to differentiate social 'facts' from social 'guesses'. Phase 2 aims to make participants better social detectives. Session 8 teaches clients about the problems in jumping to conclusions and how this is a normal cognitive event when we are unsure of the situation and others' motives. Sessions 9 and 10 involve helping the clients make better social guesses. To make this activity more concrete, 3 hypothetical characters are presented: 'My-Fault Mary' always blames herself for negative events, 'Blaming Bill' gets angry and blames others, and 'Easy Eddie' blames the situations or bad luck for negative events. These characters represent the common attributional styles present in persons with schizophrenia. Sessions 11–13 focus on separating facts from guesses. Facts are things that almost all persons will agree upon (e.g. the color of a shirt), while guesses are more open to opinion (e.g. why the persons are acting this way). Emotions are not considered facts for this exercise but guesses. To facilitate this activity, participants view pictures and videos, and come up with facts, guesses and feelings for each scene. Sessions 14 and 15 involve making better social guesses by gathering more evidence. Participants play the 20-questions game and earn points by asking yes or no questions. If they are ready to guess, they decide how many points to bet. If they are correct, they gain those points, but if they are wrong, they lose them. This exercise makes the person engage in a more deliberate decision-making process.

The primary goals of phase 3 (integration) are to assess the certainty of facts and guesses surrounding events in clients' personal lives, recognize that it is sometimes necessary to obtain more information about social situations and to teach effective social skills for checking out guesses. The purpose of the final phase is to put into practice what clients have learned in SCIT. For example, a participant arranges to go to the movies with a friend and the friend does not show up. The client then employs all of the tools learned in SCIT, such as separating facts from guesses, avoiding jumping to conclusions and gathering good data, in order to make an informed attribution for the case. The participants can then chose to check out their guess by asking the person what happened to see if their guess was correct (or ask another person or do nothing at all).

Issues to be Addressed by Future Research

Although social cognitive remediation is still in an infant stage of development, the initial efficacy results are encouraging. The existing evidence indicates that improvements in social cognitive processes essential for successful social functioning can be obtained in persons with schizophrenia by a variety of intervention approaches. As there are no direct comparisons between targeted and broad-based intervention approaches until now, the optimal treatment strategy remains unclear. However, it seems already evident that standard neurocognitive training alone is neither necessary nor sufficient to improve social cognitive processes [63].

Regardless of intervention type (cognitive versus social cognitive), there are several methodological and conceptual issues that future research needs to address. First, what is the role of social cognition in fostering improved social functioning? Research has suggested that social cognition may act as a direct predictor, mediator or moderator of social functioning. Also, social cognition can be viewed as an outcome variable related to social functioning and may not be an intervening variable at all. Thus, how distinct are social functioning and social cognition? This is important because if social cognition is believed to be a direct independent predictor, then interventions might be better served to focus on social cognitive activities instead of cognitive improvement. Most cognitive remediation studies are based on the mediator/moderator approach, with cognition being of primary importance, and its effect is exerted through social cognition to improve the person's quality of life. Second, interventions need to generalize to not only social and community functioning, but also measures and constructs not used or trained in the study. Repeated training generally improves the measures chosen in the study, but is more difficult to show improvement on novel measures, which asks an interesting question as to what is actually occurring in these treatments. Are the results simply a practice effect, or are we teaching a strategy that can be used in other situations, or perhaps we are showing the persons how to compensate for their deficits and making them more efficient? Third, improvements need to demonstrate stability over time, and surprisingly, there are very little data on the long-term effects of cognitive and social cognitive training. Finally, how many sessions are need to produce change and at what dose? It is widely known that existing treatments are costly in terms of both staff and resources, time consuming, and draining on both staff and clients. Measuring the outcome at each phase of treatment would help demonstrate the most crucial aspects of each treatment, which is similar to dismantling designs in single-subject research.

In conclusion, now that we know that social cognitive impairments are modifiable in principle, it appears worth pursuing continued development of such interventions. In order to promote functional recovery in individuals suffering from schizophrenia, future studies need to also address the translation of improvement in social cognition into broader concepts of real-life social functioning, independent living and quality of life.

References

1 Penn DL, Corrigan PW, Bentall RP, Racenstein JM, Newman L: Social cognition in schizophrenia. Psychol Bull 1997;121:114–132.

2 Penn DL, Sanna LJ, Roberts DL: Social cognition in schizophrenia: an overview. Schizophr Bull 2008;34:408–411.

3 Brothers L: The social brain: a project for integrating primate behavior and neurophysiology in a new domain. Concepts Neurosci 1990:27–61.

4 Adolphs R: The neurobiology of social cognition. Curr Opin Neurobiol 2001;11:231–239.

5 Green MF, Leitman DI: Social cognition in schizophrenia. Schizophr Bull 2008;34:670–672.

6 Penn DL, Addington J, Pinkham A: Social cognitive impairments. Am Psychiatr Publ Press 2006:261–274.

7 Pinkham AE, Penn DL, Perkins DO, Lieberman J: Implications for the neural basis of social cognition for the study of schizophrenia. Am J Psychiatry 2003;160:815–824.

8 Blackwood NJ, Howard RJ, Bentall RP, Murray RM: Cognitive neuropsychiatric models of persecutory delusions. Am J Psychiatry 2001;158:527–539.

9 Van Hooren S, Versmissen D, Janssen I, Myin-Germeys I, à Campo J, Mengelers R, van Os J, Krabbendam L: Social cognition and neurocognition as independent domains in psychosis. Schizophr Res 2008;103:257–265.

10 Sergi MJ, Rassovsky Y, Widmark C, Reist C, Erhart S, Braff DL, Marder SR, Green MF: Social cognition in schizophrenia: relationships with neurocognition and negative symptoms. Schizophr Res 2007;90:316–324.

11 Addington J, Addington D: Facial affect recognition and information processing in schizophrenia and bipolar disorder. Schizophr Res 1998;32:171–181.

12 Wölwer W, Streit M, Polzer U, Gaebel W: Facial affect recognition in the course of schizophrenia. Eur Arch Psychiatry Clin Neurosci 1996;246:165–170.

13 Couture S, Penn DL, Roberts DL: The functional significance of social cognition in schizophrenia: a review. Schizophr Bull 2006;32(suppl 1):S44–S63.

14 Bell MD, Tsang HW, Greig TC, Bryson GJ: Neurocognition, social cognition, perceived social discomfort, and vocational outcomes in schizophrenia. Schizophr Bull 2009;35:738–747.

15 Bora E, Eryavuz A, Kayahan B, Sungu G, Veznedaroglu B: Social functioning, theory of mind and neurocognition in outpatients with schizophrenia; mental state decoding may be a better predictor of social functioning than mental state reasoning. Psychiatry Res 2006;145:95–103.

16 Brüne M: Emotion recognition, 'theory of mind,' and social behavior in schizophrenia. Psychiatry Res 2005;133:135–147.

17 Pan Y, Chen S, Chen W, Liu S: Affect recognition as an independent social function determinant in schizophrenia. Comprehensive Psychiatry 2009;50:443–452.

18 Addington J, Saeedi H, Addington D: Facial affect recognition: a mediator between cognitive and social functioning in psychosis? Schizophr Res 2006;85:142–150.

19 Vauth R, Rusch N, Wirtz M, Corrigan PW: Does social cognition influence the relation between neurocognitive deficits and vocational functioning in schizophrenia? Psychiatry Res 2004;128:155–165.

20 Nienow TM, Docherty NM, Cohen AS, Dinzeo TJ: Attentional dysfunction, social perception, and social competence: what is the nature of the relationship? J Abnorm Psychol 2006;115:408–417.

21 Penn DL, Spaulding W, Reed D, Sullivan M: The relationship of social cognition to ward behavior in chronic schizophrenia. Schizophr Res 1996;20:327–335.

22 Pinkham AE, Penn DL: Neurocognitive and social cognitive predictors of interpersonal skill in schizophrenia. Psychiatry Res 2006;143:167–178.

23 Roncone R, Falloon IR, Mazza M, De Risio A, Pollice R, Necozione S, Morosini P, Casacchia M: Is theory of mind in schizophrenia more strongly associated with clinical and social functioning than with neurocognitive deficits? Psychopathology 2002;35:280–288.

24 Kuipers E, Garety P, Fowler D, Freeman D, Dunn G, Bebbington P: Cognitive, emotional, and social processes in psychosis: refining cognitive behavioral therapy for persistent positive symptoms. Schizophr Bull 2006;32(suppl 1):S24–S31.

25 Pfammatter M, Junghan UM, Brenner HD: Efficacy of psychological therapy in schizophrenia: conclusions from meta-analyses. Schizophr Bull 2006; 32(suppl 1):S64–S80.

26 Wykes T, Steel C, Everitt B, Tarrier N: Cognitive behavior therapy for schizophrenia: effect sizes, clinical models, and methodological rigor. Schizophr Bull 2008;34:523–537.

27 Moritz S, Woodward TS: Metacognitive training in schizophrenia: from basic research to knowledge translation and intervention. Curr Opin Psychiatry 2007;20:619–625.

28 Kayser N, Sarfati Y, Besche C, Hardy-Bayle MC: Elaboration of a rehabilitation method based on a pathogenetic hypothesis of 'theory of mind' impairment in schizophrenia. Neuropsychol Rehabil 2006; 16:83–95.

29 Sarfati Y, Passerieux C, Hardy-Bayle M: Can verbalization remedy the theory of mind deficit in schizophrenia? Psychopathology 2000;33:246–251.

30 Penn DL, Combs D: Modification of affect perception deficits in schizophrenia. Schizophr Res 2000; 46:217–229.

31 Combs DR, Tosheva A, Penn DL, Basso MR, Wanner JL, Laib K: Attentional shaping as a means to improve emotion perception deficits in schizophrenia. Schizophr Res 2008;105:68–77.

32 Loughland CM, Williams LM, Gordon E: Visual scan paths to positive and negative facial emotions in an outpatient schizophrenia sample. Schizophr Res 2002;55:159–170.

33 Streit M, Wölwer W, Gaebel W: Facial affect recognition and visual scanning behaviour in the course of schizophrenia. Schizophr Res 1997;24:311–317.

34 Russell TA, Chu E, Phillips ML: A pilot study to investigate the effectiveness of emotion recognition remediation in schizophrenia using the micro-expression training tool. Br J Clin Psychol 2006;45:579–583.

35 Russell TA, Green MJ, Simpson I, Coltheart M: Remediation of facial emotion perception in schizophrenia: concomitant changes in visual attention. Schizophr Res 2008;103:248–256.

36 Silver H, Goodman C, Knoll G, Isakov V: Brief emotion training improves recognition of facial emotions in chronic schizophrenia: a pilot study. Psychiatry Res 2004;128:147–154.

37 Frommann N, Streit M, Wölwer W: Remediation of facial affect recognition impairments in patients with schizophrenia: a new training program. Psychiatry Res 2003;117:281–284.

38 Wölwer W, Frommann N, Halfmann S, Piaszek A, Streit M, Gaebel W: Remediation of impairments in facial affect recognition in schizophrenia: efficacy and specificity of a new training program. Schizophr Res 2005;80:295–303.

39 Wölwer W, Frommann N: The training of affect recognition (TAR): efficacy, functional specificity, and generalization of effects. Schizophr Bull 2009;35: 351.

40 Wykes T, Reeder C, Corner J, Williams C, Everitt B: A randomised control trial of individual neurocognitive remediation: the effects on cognitive deficits and general functioning. Schizophr Res 1998;29: 164 (abstr).

41 Wilson BA, Baddeley A, Evans J, Shiel A: Errorless learning in the rehabilitation of memory-impaired people. Neuropsychol Rehabil 1994;4:307–326.

42 Ekman P, Friesen WV: Pictures of Facial Affect. Palo Alto, Consulting Psychologists Press, 1976.

43 Roder V, Mueller DR, Mueser KT, Brenner HD: Integrated psychological therapy (IPT) for schizophrenia: is it effective? Schizophr Bull 2006;32(suppl 1): S81–S93.

44 Wykes T, van der Gaag M: Is it time to develop a new cognitive therapy for psychosis – cognitive remediation therapy (CRT)? Clin Psychol Rev 2001; 21:1227–1256.

45 Hodel B, Kern RS, Brenner HD: Emotion management training (EMT) in persons with treatment-resistant schizophrenia: first results. Schizophr Res 2004;68:107–108.

46 Horan WP, Kern RS, Green MF, Penn DL: Social cognition training for individuals with schizophrenia: emerging evidence. Am J Psychiatr Rehabil 2009;11: 205–252.

47 Van der Gaag M, Kern RS, van den Bosch RJ, Liberman RP: A controlled trial of cognitive remediation in schizophrenia. Schizophr Bull 2002;28: 167–176.

48 Hodel B, Zanello A, Welling A, Mueller-Szer R, Sandner M, Wohlwend A, Wechsler Y: Ein Trainingsprogramm zur Bewältigung von maladaptiven Emotionen bei schizophren Erkrankten. Psychother Psychiatr 1997:86–89.

49 Hodel B, Brenner HD, Merlo MCG, Teuber JF: Emotional management therapy in early psychosis. Br J Psychiatry 1998;172:128–133.

50 Hogarty GE, Flesher S, Ulrich R, Carter M, Greenwald D, Pogue-Geile M, Kechavan M, Cooley S, DiBarry AL, Garrett A, Parepally H, Zoretich R: Cognitive enhancement therapy for schizophrenia: effects of a 2-year randomized trial on cognition and behavior. Arch Gen Psychiatry 2004;61:866–876.

51 Eack SM, Hogarty GE, Greenwald DP, Hogarty SS, Keshavan MS: Cognitive enhancement therapy improves emotional intelligence in early course schizophrenia: preliminary effects. Schizophr Res 2007;89: 308–311.

52 Mayer JD, Salovey P, Caruso DR, Sitarenios G: Measuring emotional intelligence with the MSCEIT V2.0. Emotion 2003;3:97–105.

53 Vauth R, Joe A, Seitz M, Dreher-Rudolph M, Olbrich H, Stieglitz RD: Differentiated short- and long-term effects of a 'training of emotional intelligence' and of the 'integrated psychologic therapy program' for schizophrenic patients? FortschriNeurol Psychiatr 2001;69:518–525.

54 Choi KH, Kwon JH: Social cognition enhancement training for schizophrenia: a preliminary randomized controlled trial. Community Ment Health J 2006;42:177–187.

55 Combs DR, Adams SD, Penn DL, Roberts D, Tiegreen J, Stem P: Social cognition and interaction training (SCIT) for inpatients with schizophrenia spectrum disorders: preliminary findings. Schizophr Res 2007;91:112–116.

56 Penn D, Roberts DL, Munt ED, Silverstein E, Jones N, Sheitman B: A pilot study of social cognition and interaction training (SCIT) for schizophrenia. Schizophr Res 2005;80:357–359.

57 Roberts DL, Penn DL: Social cognition and interaction training (SCIT) for outpatients with schizophrenia: a preliminary study. Psychiatry Res 2009; 166:141–147.

58 Turner-Brown LM, Perry TD, Dichter GS, Bodfish JW, Penn DL: Brief report: feasibility of social cognition and interaction training for adults with high-functioning autism. J Autism Dev Disord 2008;38: 1777–1784.

59 Combs DR, Penn DL, Tiegreen JA, Nelson A, Ledet SN, Basso MR, Elerson K: Stability and generalization of social cognition and interaction training (SCIT) for schizophrenia: six-month follow-up results. Schizophr Res 2009;112:196–197.

60 Horan WP, Kern RS, Shokat-Fadai K, Sergi MJ, Wynn JK, Green MF: Social cognitive skills training in schizophrenia: an initial efficacy study of stabilized outpatients. Schizophr Res 2009;107:47–54.

61 Roberts DL, Penn DL, Combs DL: Social Cognition and Interaction Training Manual. Unpublished manuscript, 2006.

62 Penn DL, Roberts DL, Combs D, Sterne A: Best practices: the development of the social cognition and interaction training program for schizophrenia spectrum disorders. Psychiatr Serv 2007;58:449–451.

63 Kern RS, Glynn SM, Horan WP, Marder SR: Psychosocial treatments to promote functional recovery in schizophrenia. Schizophr Bull 2009;35: 347–361.

Prof. Dr. Wolfgang Wölwer
Department of Psychiatry and Psychotherapy
Heinrich Heine University Düsseldorf, Rhineland State Clinics Düsseldorf
Bergische Landstrasse 2, DE–40629 Düsseldorf (Germany)
Tel. +49 211 922 2002, Fax +49 211 922 2020, E-Mail woelwer@uni-duesseldorf.de

Roder V, Medalia A (eds): Neurocognition and Social Cognition in Schizophrenia Patients. Basic Concepts and Treatment. Key Issues Ment Health. Basel, Karger, 2010, vol 177, pp 79–84

4.1

Training of Emotional Intelligence in Schizophrenia

Roland Vauth

Psychiatrische Poliklinik, Universitätsspital Basel, Basel, Switzerland

Abstract

Training microskills of emotional intelligence may be a promising opportunity to improve functional recovery in schizophrenia. The chapter details the different components of emotional intelligence and discusses its relevance in the treatment of schizophrenia. The modules of a published training program are characterized with some clinical details.   Copyright © 2010 S. Karger AG, Basel

Aspects of Emotional Intelligence: Bridging the Gap between Remission and Functional Recovery?

Since functional recovery in schizophrenia is rare in spite of successful controlling of positive symptoms [1], it is useful to explore the particular barriers of treatment and rehabilitation [2]. Cognitive deficits and negative symptoms have clearly been shown to limit treatment and rehabilitation readiness, thus the ability to benefit from interventions. Nevertheless, cognitive dysfunctions, that is, nonsocial information-processing deficits, appear to have only a limited predictive value for social functioning [3, 4]. In contrast, appropriate processing of socioemotional information has a greater external validity and provides an improved understanding of the patient's social competencies and problems in everyday life [2, 5, 6].

Since the time of Eugen Bleuler emotional processing deficits have been regarded as a core feature of dysfunction in schizophrenia that is independent of the cultural background. Deficits in facial affect recognition are well established [7]. The relevance of emotion recognition as a predictor of functional outcome has been well documented [8, 9]. In the following, we illustrate the relevance and implications of specific socioemotional competencies for schizophrenia and discuss them in a framework of emotional intelligence to derive appropriate intervention strategies.

There are 2 main reasons to address socioemotional information-processing deficits in patients with schizophrenia. Firstly, emotional processing deficits may represent 'rate-limiting factors' for psychosocial function and response rate to psychosocial interventions [2]. Cognitive behavioral interventions may thus enhance the patient's readiness for rehabilitation and social functioning within the community. Secondly, since emotional information-processing deficits play an important role in stress vulnerability, a reduction in such deficits may be an appropriate strategy for general relapse prevention [10].

In spite of the importance of social cognition and emotional processing in schizophrenia, less emphasis has been placed upon the improvement of socioemotional skills. Recently, however, training programs have been developed to address the issue of socioemotional skills and behavior [11–13]. The Integrated Psychological Therapy for Schizophrenia [14–16] emphasizes general cognitive capabilities but also encompasses training of social skills as well as social perception. Cognitive Enhancement Therapy [17] is one of the few attempts to address both social information processing and cognitive deficits.

Training of Emotional Intelligence: The Treatment Rationale

Due to growing evidence suggesting that social cognition and emotional processing skills may influence role functioning [2, 6], some approaches directly focus on this set of functions. We have previously developed a training program of emotional intelligence for schizophrenia [13, 18]. This approach has been introduced within the emotional intelligence framework of Salovey et al. [19, 20]. The first 3 factors (emotional perception, emotional understanding and emotional management) constitute the basis of this training program because emotional self-perception, perception of others and shifting to another perspective were found to compromise social problem solving and empathy in schizophrenia [21–24].

The ability to understand emotional information was specifically impaired in schizophrenia. Problems in emotional perspective taking co-occurred with emotional comprehension and reasoning deficits [25]. Emotional management also aims at mood regulation deficits in schizophrenia [10]. It is a well-accepted fact that persons with schizophrenia tend to cope with negative emotions and stress in a relatively avoidant and ineffectual manner like passive avoidant strategies and reduced reliance on active problem solving and poor social support seeking [26, 27].

Emotional reactivity and subsequent higher stress responsiveness has been demonstrated to be more pronounced in schizophrenia [28]. As higher reactivity to emotional stress was found to be related to the disposition to experience intense aversive emotional states and to a lower tendency to experience positive or rewarding emotional states [29], our program focuses on both coping with negative emotions as well as on the ability to maintain positive emotional states.

Modules and Components of the Training of Emotional Intelligence in Schizophrenia

The training schedule consists of 12 sessions during a 6-week period. Two 80-min sessions per week are administered to patient groups with a mean size of 6–8 participants. In each session, 3 basic components are realized (emotional perception, emotional understanding and emotional management). These target areas are mostly treated in parallel but with different emphases. Therapist and patient workbooks have been developed for each session and a treatment manual was published more recently [30]. In the first part of the session, skills related to the perception and interpretation of emotion information are trained. The focus of the second part of each training session is emotional management, that is, to enhance the capacity to self-regulate emotions.

Component 1: Perception and Interpretation of Emotions

Discrimination Tasks
Patients are requested to distinguish different emotions (Ekman and Friesen series of facial affect expressions). Usually, 2 pictures are presented to show the difference between the emotional states of the depicted stimulus persons.

Matching Tasks
First, the patient is asked to compare facial affect recognition pictures with his inferences concerning the core emotions of the stimulus person in a written short story (e.g. situations of loss, threat or enjoyment). Secondly, to improve self-perception of emotional states, affect recognition and shared feelings are addressed by asking the patients to select 1 or 2 pictures or objects (e.g. different postcards, scarves or small stones) presented on a table, which may reflect their current mood. The patient is requested to explain the picture to the group (training of emotional expression). The participants are further encouraged to explore whether other group members who validate the emotional meaning are aware of their own feelings and are able to share these with others (training of emotional perspective taking). These perception tasks may also be regarded as activation exercises (motivation and promotion of cognitive receptiveness).

Training of Social Inferences and Reasoning in Affective Social Situations
This section focuses on emotional understanding. Written short stories describing situations of loss, threat or enjoyment are given and questions are asked, such as: 'Describe what was going on.' 'Why do you think that . . .?' 'What is the evidence for supposing that . . .?' 'What do you think, would be the consequence of . . .?'

Behavioral Analyses

Behavioral analyses are intended to support the development and consolidation of emotional reasoning processes. Here, 2 patients are requested to interview each other ('reporter exercise') concerning internal or external stimuli that may elicit specific emotional responses.

Component 2: Self-Regulation of Emotions

The strategies trained in the second part of each session include coping with negative affective states such as depression (sessions 1–3) and anxiety (sessions 4–6). In the following sessions, specific strategies for maintaining positive emotional states (sessions 7–9) and developing interests and initiative (sessions 10–12) are elaborated.

The emotional management section starts with a *psychoeducational phase* that provides a rationale for enhancing coping skills for a particular target emotion which aims at both relapse prevention and everyday functioning. The importance of the specific target emotion is elaborated interactively for the participants (e.g. disengagement of therapy or rehabilitation and depression). The role of negative emotion as a destabilizing factor or as a prodromal symptom of an emerging relapse and of positive emotion as a protective factor is discussed. Situational models of individual 'vicious circles' (emotion-perception-interpretation-action) are elaborated and 'exit' strategies are discussed. Moreover, the neurobiological rationale of pharmacological treatment of negative emotions such as depression and anxiety is provided.

In the following 2 sessions on each target emotion, this knowledge is individually applied. The aim is to improve coping with negative emotions in subjectively relevant social and job-related situations. Personal triggers of negative feelings are elaborated.

Self-recording corresponding to the *ABC scheme* (i.e. recording of the activating event, of beliefs and automatic thoughts and of the consequences) is applied to situations that are experienced as stressful by the individual. Exploring internal and external cues of the respective target emotion and identifying coping strategies is trained by role reversal in a *'reporter' exercise*: 'You said that you are depressed after. . . .' 'What did you think about this?' 'How did you try to feel better?' The results are presented to the group, and the other participants are requested to make suggestions how to cope more efficiently with the situation.

This section aims at replacing dysfunctional coping strategies such as alcohol and drug consumption or social withdrawal with more efficient techniques. These methods of appropriate self-management are enhanced by *modeling and rehearsal of additional coping strategies* (such as relaxation techniques, identification and challenge of dysfunctional thoughts, distracting and focusing strategies). Supported by the therapist, each patient chooses a maximum of 3 coping strategies and records them on 'coping cards' that are kept in a pocket or posted in the patient's private environment. The patient is encouraged to read them regularly (e.g. 3 times a day). These cards may have several forms such as writing a central automatic thought or belief on one side and its adaptive response on the other, devising behavioral strategies for specific problem situations or arranging activating self-instructions.

The session devoted to the *promotion of positive feelings* involves an elaboration of individual strategies for emotional self-control. The patient learns to apply various techniques to promote positive feelings, to systematically plan positive activities (pleasure technique), to use self-reinforcement or to plan periods of enjoyment. In sessions 10–12, strategies for an appropriate leisure time planning are developed on the level of the individual. Already existing strategies and behaviors such as the identification of significant reinforcers and their contingent use are also promoted. As an effect of cognitive enhancement therapy, an improved understanding and managing of one's own and others' emotions could be demonstrated [17].

References

1 Robinson DG, Woerner MG, McMeniman M, Mendelowitz A, Bilder RM: Symptomatic and functional recovery from a first episode of schizophrenia or schizoaffective disorder. Am J Psychiatry 2004; 161:473–479.

2 Vauth R, Rüsch N, Wirtz M, Corrigan PW: Does social cognition influence the relation between neurocognitive deficits and vocational functioning in schizophrenia? Psychiatry Res 2004;128:155–165.

3 Barch DM: The relationships among cognition, motivation, and emotion in schizophrenia: how much and how little we know. Schizophr Bull 2005; 31:875–881.

4 Hooker C, Park S: Emotion processing and its relationship to social functioning in schizophrenia patients. Psychiatry Res 2002;112:41–50.

5 Bell M, Tsang HW, Greig TC, Bryson GJ: Neurocognition, social cognition, perceived social discomfort, and vocational outcomes in schizophrenia. Schizophr Bull 2008;35:378–747.

6 Penn DL, Corrigan PW, Bentall RP, Racenstein JM, Newman L: Social cognition in schizophrenia. Psychol Bull 1997;121:114–132.

7 Sachs G, Steger-Wuchse D, Kryspin-Exner I, Gur RC, Katschnig H: Facial recognition deficits and cognition in schizophrenia. Schizophr Res 2004;68: 27–35.

8 Hall J, Harris JM, Sprengelmeyer R, Sprengelmeyer A, Young AW, Santos IM, Johnstone EC, Lawrie SM: Social cognition and face processing in schizophrenia. Br J Psychiatry 2004;185:169–170.

9 Phillips ML: Facial processing deficits and social dysfunction: how are they related? Brain 2004;127: 1691–1692.

10 Horan WP, Blanchard JJ: Neurocognitive, social, and emotional dysfunction in deficit syndrome schizophrenia. Schizophr Res 2003;65:125–137.

11 Hogarty GE, Flesher S, Ulrich R, Carter M, Greenwald D, Pogue-Geile M, Kechavan M, Cooley S, Dibarry AL, Garrett A, Parepally H, Zoretich R: Cognitive enhancement therapy for schizophrenia: effects of a 2-year randomized trial on cognition and behavior. Arch Gen Psychiatry 2004;61:866–876.

12 Penn DL, Combs DR, Ritchie M, Francis J, Cassisi J, Morris S, Townsend M: Emotion recognition in schizophrenia: further investigation of generalized versus specific deficit models. J Abnorm Psychol 2000;109:512–516.

13 Vauth R, Joe A, Seitz M, Dreher-Rudolph M, Olbrich H, Stieglitz RD: Differenzielle Kurz- und Langzeitwirkung eines 'Trainings Emotionaler Intelligenz' und des 'Integrierten Psychologischen Therapieprogramms' für schizophrene Patienten. Fortschr Neurol Psychiatr 2001;69:518–525.

14 Hodel B, Kern RS, Brenner HD: Emotion Management Training (EMT) in persons with treatment-resistant schizophrenia: first results. Schizophr Res 2004;68:107–108.

15 Roder V, Müller DR, Mueser KT, Brenner HD: The effectiveness of Integrated Psychological Therapy (IPT) for schizophrenia patients: a meta-analysis covering 30 independent studies. Schizophr Bull 2006;32:S81–S93.

16 Roder V, Mueller D, Spaulding W, Brenner HD: Integrated Psychological Therapy for Schizophrenia Patients (IPT). Goettingen, Hogrefe, 2010.

17 Eack SM, Hogarty GE, Greenwald DP, Hogarty SS, Keshavan MS: Cognitive enhancement therapy improves emotional intelligence in early course schizophrenia: preliminary effects. Schizophr Res 2007;89: 308–311.

18 Vauth R, Dreher-Rudolph M, Ueber R, Olbrich HM: Das 'Training Emotionaler Intelligenz'. Ein neuer Therapieansatz in der Gruppenpsychotherapie schizophrener Patienten; in Mundt C, Linden M, Barnett W (eds): Psychotherapie in der Psychiatrie. New York, Springer, 1997, pp 87–91.

19 Mayer JD, Caruso DR, Salovey P: Emotional intelligence meets traditional standards for an intelligence. Intelligence 2000;27:267–298.

20 Mayer JD, Salovey P, Caruso D: Competing models of emotional intelligence; in Sternberg RJ (ed): Handbook of Human Intelligence. New York, Cambridge University Press, 2001.

21 Mueser KT: Schizophrenia; in Bellack AS, Hersen M (eds): Handbook of Behavior Therapy in the Psychiatric Setting. New York, Plenum Press, 1993, pp 260–291.

22 Shamay-Tsoory SG, Shur S, Barcai-Goodman L, Medlovich S, Harari H, Levkovitz Y: Dissociation of cognitive from affective components of theory of mind in schizophrenia. Psychiatry Res 2007;149:11–23.

23 Shamay-Tsoory SG, Shur S, Harari H, Levkovitz Y: Neurocognitive basis of impaired empathy in schizophrenia. Neuropsychology 2007;21:431–438.

24 Vollm BA, Taylor AN, Richardson P, Corcoran R, Stirling J, McKie S, Deakin JF, Elliott R: Neuronal correlates of theory of mind and empathy: a functional magnetic resonance imaging study in a nonverbal task. Neuroimage 2006;29:90–98.

25 Greig TC, Bryson GJ, Bell MD: Theory of mind performance in schizophrenia: diagnostic, symptom, and neuropsychological correlates. J Nerv Ment Dis 2004;192:12–18.

26 Lancaster RS, Evans JD, Bond GR, Lysaker PH: Social cognition and neurocognitive deficits in schizophrenia. J Nerv Ment Dis 2003;191:295–299.

27 Lysaker PH, Campbell K, Johannesen JK: Hope, awareness of illness, and coping in schizophrenia spectrum disorders: evidence of an interaction. J Nerv Ment Dis 2005;193:287–292.

28 Cohen AS, Docherty NM: Affective reactivity of speech and emotional experience in patients with schizophrenia. Schizophr Res 2004;69:7–14.

29 Berenbaum H, Williams M: Personality and emotional reactivity. J Res Pers 1995;29:24–34.

30 Vauth R, Stieglitz RD: Das Training Emotionaler Intelligenz bei schizophrenen Störungen. Soziale Kognition und emotionale Verarbeitung im Fokus erfolgreicher Rehabilitation. Göttingen, Hogrefe, 2008.

Priv.-Doz. Dr. med. Dipl.-Psych. Roland Vauth
Psychiatrische Poliklinik, Universitätsspital Basel
Claragraben 95
CH–4005 Basel (Switzerland)
Tel. +41 61 699 25 25, Fax +41 61 699 25 25, E-Mail rvauth@uhbs.ch

Roder V, Medalia A (eds): Neurocognition and Social Cognition in Schizophrenia Patients. Basic Concepts and Treatment. Key Issues Ment Health. Basel, Karger, 2010, vol 177, pp 85–103

5
_____

Combined Treatment Approaches: Overview and Empirical Results

Volker Roder[a] · Lea Hulka[a] · Alice Medalia[b]

[a]University Hospital of Psychiatry Bern, Bern, Switzerland; [b]Department of Psychiatry, Columbia University College of Physicians and Surgeons, New York, N.Y., USA

_____

Abstract

This chapter provides an overview of existing combined treatment approaches that aim at enhancing neurocognitive and social cognitive functioning in patients with schizophrenia and schizoaffective disorder. The approaches discussed are the Integrated Psychological Therapy (IPT), the Integrated Neurocognitive Therapy (INT), the Cognitive Enhancement Therapy (CET), the Neurocognitive Enhancement Therapy (NET) and the Neuropsychological Educational Approach to Cognitive Remediation (NEAR). Altogether, corresponding empirical efficacy studies indicate that all the reviewed treatment approaches significantly contribute to improvement in functional outcome and recovery in schizophrenia. A question that remains open concerns the influence of group processes on improvement in significant areas. Future research should focus on clarifying underlying effectiveness mechanisms of group treatments.   Copyright © 2010 S. Karger AG, Basel

In this chapter combined treatment approaches and corresponding empirical results are reviewed. Combined treatment approaches, also referred to as integrative approaches, aim at improving both neurocognitive and social cognitive functioning. In general, interventions to target cognitive impairments can either be 'cognition enhancing' and designed to improve cognitive functions (e.g. repetitive exercises) or 'compensatory', seeking to bypass or compensate cognitive deficits (e.g. strategies to organize information). Interventions to target social cognition focus on components such as emotion perception, social perception, theory of mind and attributional bias. In addition, combined treatment approaches may contain elements of social skill training targeting impaired behavior in occupational, social and recreational situations [1].

Over the past 4 decades, several neurocognitive and social cognitive rehabilitation approaches have been developed. In the following, their historical development is briefly outlined. In the 1970s, the Integrated Psychological Therapy (IPT) [2] was

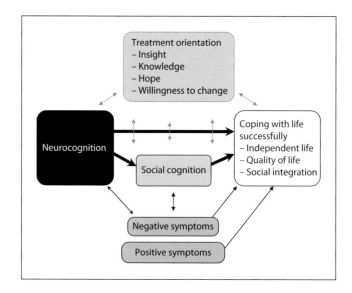

Fig. 1. Mediating variables between neurocognition and functional outcome [2, 11].

introduced and served as a predecessor for subsequent programs. For example, the Cognitive Enhancement Therapy (CET) and the Cognitive Remediation Therapy [3–6] were influenced by IPT, and the very recently conceptualized Integrated Neurocognitive Therapy (INT) [7] is a direct further development of IPT. Later emerging approaches were able to rely on already existing knowledge as well as to expedite their own developments. For instance, the Neuropsychological Educational Approach to Cognitive Remediation (NEAR) [8] strongly acknowledges the importance of intrinsic motivation in patients, and the Neurocognitive Enhancement Therapy (NET) [9] has a special focus on work rehabilitation.

Most of the combined treatment approaches have a reference to or are based on integrative recovery models of functional outcome and recovery [10]. One of the most influential ones is the model originally proposed by Green and Nuechterlein [11]. They postulated that the relationship between neurocognition and functional outcome is at least partially mediated by social cognition. A number of studies using structural equation modeling have provided empirical evidence for this assumption [12–16]. Moreover, in recent years, further mediating and moderating variables that are crucial for functional outcome have been identified, as is depicted in figure 1.

A considerable body of research suggests that the individual treatment orientation of patients comprising variables such as insight into illness [17], extrinsic and intrinsic motivation [18–20], empowerment, hope and knowledge [21, 22] significantly affects successful recovery. Hence both neurocognition and social cognition as well as treatment orientation are important intervention targets.

Several meta-analyses regarding neurocognitive and social cognitive remediation have been conducted [23–28]. Overall, moderate range effect sizes (ES) are found for

Roder · Hulka · Medalia

Table 1. Findings of the meta-analyses concerning the effects of neurocognitive and social cognitive remediation

Meta-analysis	Outcome variable	Effect size
Kurtz et al. [23], 2001 (11 CT)	executive functioning	0.98
Krabbendam and Aleman [25], 2003 (12 CT)	cognitive functioning	0.45
Twamley et al. [26], 2003 (17 CT)	cognitive functioning	0.32
	social functioning	0.51
	general psychopathology	0.26
Pilling et al. [35], 2002 (5 RCT)	attention	0.11
	verbal memory	0.14
	visual memory	0.34
	general psychopathology	0.23
Pfammatter et al. [27], 2006 (19 RCT)	attention	0.32
	memory	0.36
	executive functioning	0.28
	social cognition	0.40
	social functioning	0.49
	general psychopathology	0.20
	negative symptoms	0.24
McGurk et al. [28], 2007 (26 RCT)	global cognition	0.41
	attention/vigilance	0.41
	speed of processing	0.48
	verbal working memory	0.52
	verbal learning and memory	0.39
	visual learning and memory	0.09
	reasoning/problem solving	0.47
	social cognition	0.54
	symptoms	0.28
	functioning	0.35

CT = Controlled trial; RCT = randomized controlled trial.

the impact of behavioral treatment on neurocognition and social cognition, as can be seen in table 1.

With the exception of Pilling et al. [24], who only reviewed a small and highly selected set of studies, reviews have reported mostly beneficial effects. Furthermore, there is evidence for beneficial effects on psychosocial functioning. For example, McGurk et al. [28], in their meta-analysis of 26 randomized controlled trials of cognitive remediation in schizophrenia, reported a medium ES for cognitive performance, a slightly lower level of psychosocial functioning and a small ES for symptoms. It is noteworthy that the effects of cognitive remediation therapy on psychosocial functioning were significantly greater in studies that included participation in adjunctive rehabilitation programs than those with cognitive remediation alone.

The American Psychological Association Committee for the Advancement of Professional Practice has listed 8 evidence-based approaches to cognitive remediation in the '2007 training grid outlining best practices for recovery and improved outcomes for people with serious mental illness' [30]. These approaches are the attention process training by Sohlberg and Mateer, the IPT by Roder et al., the CET by Hogarty et al., the NET by Bell, the cognitive remediation therapy by Delahunty and Wykes, the NEAR by Medalia and Revheim, the errorless learning approaches by Kern as well as attention shaping by Silverstein and Menditto. In the following, the currently available combined therapy approaches, constituting the state of the art in this emerging field, that target both neurocognitive and social cognitive functioning shall be presented as well as corresponding empirical data regarding their effectiveness. In addition, the INT will also be described, as it is a direct further development of IPT. Treatment approaches that specifically target neurocognition or social cognition alone are discussed in chapters 3 and 4.

Integrated Psychological Therapy (IPT)

IPT was one of the first systematically structured, comprehensive and manualized treatment approaches that were specifically designed for the rehabilitation of schizophrenia patients [2]. IPT is a cognitive behavioral therapy program that combines neurocognitive and social cognitive interventions with social skill approaches with the end goal of improving social competence. According to IPT, basic deficits in neurocognitive functioning exert negative effects on higher-order behavioral functions, including social skills, social functioning and independent functioning [31]. Based on this assumption, in order to achieve successful psychosocial rehabilitation, both underlying neurocognitive and social cognitive impairments as well as social, self-care and vocational skills need to be remediated. IPT is structured into 5 subprograms with increasing levels of complexity that are taught sequentially as a building-block model is postulated. The first subprogram, 'cognitive differentiation', aims at enhancing neurocognitive functioning (e.g. attention, verbal memory, cognitive flexibility, concept formation). The second subprogram, 'social perception', targets social cognitive deficits (e.g. social and emotional perception, emotional expression). The third subprogram, 'verbal communication', addresses verbal fluency and executive functioning, thus skills that impact interpersonal communication directly. Moreover, it constitutes the link between the more cognitively oriented first 2 subprograms and the more behaviorally oriented last 2 subprograms. The fourth, 'social skills', and the fifth, 'interpersonal problem-solving', subprograms foster building social competence through the development of interpersonal skills by means of role plays and through group-based problem-solving exercises. Therapy is guided by a well-trained therapist and a cotherapist and takes place in small groups comprising 5–8 participants in 30- to 60-min sessions 3 times per week over a 6-month period. In addition, in vivo exercises and homework assignments as well as individualized sessions by request of patients or therapists are implemented. Meanwhile, IPT has been widely adopted, particularly in Europe, but also in North America and Asia. Currently, the sixth edition of the German manual is available [32] and translations into 12 other languages [33].

IPT Efficacy Studies

Over the past 25 years, IPT was evaluated in 34 studies with 1,515 patients conducted by research groups in 12 different countries. Roder et al. [modified from 33, 34] integrated these results in a meta-analysis that examined the efficacy of IPT. IPT was either compared with standard care (pharmacotherapy and social therapy), with a placebo-attention condition (nonspecific group activity) or with both simultaneously. In 2 studies, IPT was used as a control condition, and in 5 no control group existed. The studies had various sample sizes ranging from 17 to 143 patients, different methodological rigor in terms of randomization and blind expert ratings, included in- as well as outpatient settings, and had taken place in academic and nonacademic sites. The patient characteristics were as follows: 68% were male, with a mean age of 35 years and an IQ generally over 90. The duration and number of hospitalizations, as well as the duration of the illness and the daily dose of antipsychotic medication were largely heterogeneous. The mean treatment period was 17.2 weeks with 49.3 h and a mean frequency of 3.2 sessions per week, with earlier studies indicating a higher frequency of therapy sessions, whereas more recent ones generally administered 2-weekly sessions. The average dropout rate during the treatment period was 14.7% and 15.6% during the entire trial.

In a first step, all 34 published IPT studies were included in the meta-analysis, comprising a sample of 1,515 patients.

Of special interest were (1) *the global therapy effect,* defined as the mean of all assessed outcome variables referring to documented symptom dimensions, neurocognitive and social functioning, quality of life, well-being, as well as treatment satisfaction at the end of therapy and at follow-up; (2) *separate symptom dimensions and functional impairments*, including neurocognition (attention, memory, executive functioning), psychopathology (negative and positive symptoms) and psychosocial functioning (social and role functioning, self-care, occupational skills); (3) *singular tests* used in different studies to control the comparability of the assessments addressing different symptom and functional domains; (4) *moderators of treatment response,* including patient characteristics (e.g. gender), setting (e.g. inpatient/outpatient) and site conditions (e.g. academic and nonacademic sites), and and (5) *predictors of outcome* defined as the influence on outcome by moderating variables of patient characteristics and setting.

IPT obtained a significantly higher weighted mean effect size of 0.51 for global therapy outcome (changes from baseline to the posttreatment assessment) compared with the placebo-attention condition that exhibited a small ES of 0.24 and the groups receiving standard care 0.13. The mean ES was defined as the mean of all assessed outcome variables (symptom dimensions, neurocognitive and social functioning, quality of life, well-being and treatment satisfaction). The IPT group still obtained superior effects at an average of 8.1 months later follow-up, providing evidence for a vertical generalization. Positive mean ES favoring IPT over control groups were also found for neurocognition (0.54), psychopathology (0.50) and psychosocial functioning (0.41).

Furthermore, the effects obtained by IPT emerged to be similarly favorable across the different outcome domains of assessment format (self-rating ES = 0.51, expert rating ES = 0.48 and psychological testing ES = 0.52), settings (inpatient ES = 0.53 vs. outpatient ES = 0.49), centers (academic ES = 0.56 vs. nonacademic ES = 0.50) and state of illness (symptom-stabilized ES = 0.52 vs. postacute ES = 0.50). However, the duration of illness had a negative effect on the global therapy outcome of IPT. Thus, patients with a longer background of illness did not benefit as much from IPT. In contrast, age and duration of hospitalization had a moderate negative effect on global therapy outcome. The global therapy outcome was neither correlated with the duration of therapy, the number of therapy sessions nor with the weekly frequency of therapy sessions, but the functional outcome was improved by longer therapy duration.

In a second step, 8 high-quality studies including 401 patients and satisfying high methodological rigor, such as randomized patient allocation, blind ratings and controlled medication, were selected and corroborated the previous results obtained from the 34 studies.

A further study conducted by Mueller and Roder [34] evaluated and compared the effects of the different IPT subprograms as well as their combination. Interventions solely based on the neurocognitive subprogram 'cognitive differentiation' significantly improved the proximal outcome (ES = 0.40) but generated no significant effects for distal outcome. The combination of the neurocognitive and social cognitive IPT subprograms ('cognitive differentiation' and 'social perception'), however, obtained favorable effects for neurocognition (ES = 0.74), social cognition (ES = 0.82) as well as social functioning (ES = 0.40). Furthermore, the relapse rate of the group receiving neurocognitive therapy (22.2%) was higher than for the combined intervention group (11.8%).

In summary, the meta-analysis proved IPT to be an effective rehabilitation approach for schizophrenia that is robust across a wide range of patients and treatment conditions. The results indicate that the integration of neurocognitive rehabilitation and psychosocial skill training may work synergistically to improve both domains more effectively than either intervention alone and also may be important for the generalization of these effects to distal, thus, functional outcome. Critically stated, although IPT obtained superior effects in functional outcome compared with control groups, the effects on psychosocial functioning are usually smaller than for neurocognition and psychopathology, as has been reported in other meta-analyses [35, 24]. For more detailed information concerning the IPT see chapter 5.2.

Integrated Neurocognitive Therapy (INT)

The INT [7] is a cognitive behavioral group therapy program that constitutes a further development of the cognitive part of the IIPT. The conceptualization of INT is based on modern recovery models [e.g. 2, 11] that not only highlight the importance of enhancing psychosocial functioning in patients but also postulate that the relationship between neurocognition and functional outcome may be (partially) mediated by social cognition. Thus both neuro- and social cognition are important intervention targets, as is reflected in the main therapy goals. As a proximal goal, INT intends to restitute and compensate neurocognition and social cognitive (dys-) functions by systematically targeting the dimensions defined by the MATRICS initiative (Measurement and Treatment Research to Improve Cognition in Schizophrenia): speed of processing, attention/vigilance, verbal and visual learning and memory, working memory, reasoning and problem solving, emotional and social perception, social schema and emotion regulation [36, 37]. These domains are subsumed into 4 modules. The first modules are more structured, include more computer-based exercises, and are of less cognitive complexity and emotional strain compared to subsequent modules. As a more distal goal, INT attempts to improve neurocognitive and social cognitive functioning in the broader everyday life context, meaning that patients' psychosocial functioning ought to be ameliorated by enhancing their ability to function properly and independently within a community, by increasing their life quality and social integration in the areas of work, living and recreational activities. Furthermore, therapy in INT is embedded in a daily living context in order to facilitate transfer. In addition, a strong focus is placed on patients' resource activation so as to rear an understanding of one's own strengths and weaknesses in cognitive and social domains. Thereupon based, individualized coping strategies to optimize existing difficulties in daily life can be derived. INT also places a strong emphasis on fostering patients' intrinsic therapy motivation as well as their self-efficacy expectancy in terms of creating a sense of self-empowerment.

A therapy manual has already been developed and is currently in further progress [38]. Therapy takes place in small groups comprising 6–8 participants. A well-trained therapist and a cotherapist guide the patients through the program over a 4-month period. Sessions take place biweekly and last 90 min each (including a short break). In total, 30 sessions are administered.

The 4 modules follow the same didactic therapy components. Thus, each treatment area is structured in introductory sessions where patients are encouraged to perceive their own available resources and difficulties as well as possibilities for optimization and where psychoeducation regarding the specific treatment areas is provided (e.g. how a certain deficit may impact daily functioning). Educational information is usually presented in case vignettes that are related to situations patients are likely to encounter. In consecutive sessions compensation (generating individual coping strategies) and restitution (rehearsal) are the crucial intervention targets. With each therapy module the level of complexity and emotional strain increases, and the exercises become less structured. Whereas initially the tasks are more frequently computer based, the exercises in later modules take place in group settings with less use of computers. In addition, for all therapy components in vivo exercises and homework assignments are encouraged to promote transfer and generalization. For further information see chapter 5.2.

INT Efficacy Studies

The effectiveness of INT is currently being evaluated in an international randomized multicenter study in Switzerland, Germany and Austria [7]. INT is compared with treatment as usual (TAU), whereby patients receive 30 therapy sessions each lasting 90 min for 15 weeks. Outpatients with a schizophrenia diagnosis according to the criteria of DSM-IV-TR are included. Assessment instruments are administered before (T1) and after therapy (T2) as well as after a 1-year follow-up (T3) and measure neurocognition, social cognition, psychopathology, social functioning, quality of life, self-efficacy expectation and therapy motivation. In addition, the therapy process is evaluated through patients and therapists. All expert ratings are carried out blindly by independent raters.

The most recent patient sample comprised data for 145 patients for T1, of whom 75 were in the INT group and 70 in the TAU group, 129 (INT = 67, TAU = 62) for T2 and 113 (INT = 59, TAU = 54) for T3. During the treatment time there were 8 dropouts (11%), and during follow-up time another 8 dropped out, which constitutes a total dropout rate of 22%. The patient characteristics did not significantly differ between the 2 groups. The mean age was 35 years (SD = 9.0), the mean age at illness onset was 24 years (SD = 7.4), and the mean IQ (WIP) was around 104 standard points (SD = 9.6). Large variances were found for duration of illness, symptoms and medication. As to be expected, more men than women participated in the study (61.3% INT; 71.4% TAU). The INT group significantly improved compared to the TAU group when data obtained from baseline and after therapy were examined (pre-post) in the areas of speed of processing (RWT), attention/vigilance (d2) and emotion perception (PFA, EMOREC). In addition, the patients from the INT group showed a significant reduction in positive, negative and general symptoms (Positive and Negative Syndrome Scale), a mean value of psychopathology as well as improved social functioning (Global Assessment of Functioning Scale) after therapy. The favorable effects of the INT group were maintained except for speed of processing (RWT) and positive symptoms (Positive and Negative Syndrome Scale), and some additional improvements were found in the areas of verbal learning and memory (AVLT), as well as social attribution (AIHQ) after the 1-year follow-up phase.

As the study is ongoing, the obtained results have to be regarded as preliminary. Nevertheless, the findings imply horizontal generalization (proximal and distal outcomes are ameliorated) and vertical generalization (additional improvement after the follow-up phase) of the INT. The low dropout rate (11%) and good acceptance of patients and therapists indicate high clinical relevance of INT. Further results, especially the follow-up data, have to confirm the significance of the newly developed neurocognitive and social cognitive remediation approach.

Cognitive Enhancement Therapy (CET)

CET [39–42] is a holistic, developmental approach aiming at the rehabilitation of social cognitive and neurocognitive deficits among patients with schizophrenia and schizoaffective disorder in the postacute phase of the illness. The underlying model of CET postulates that impaired social cognition is a result of neurodevelopmental disturbances. Furthermore, it is claimed that a presumed neuroplasticity reserve can respond to enriched cognitive experiences.

The conceptualization of CET was considerably influenced by the IPT of Roder et al. [2] for schizophrenia patients and the work of Ben-Yishay et al. [43] with traumatic brain injury patients as well as a contemporary theory of human cognitive development [44].

The emphasis in training is to shift from verbatim, concrete cognitive information processing that is characteristic of earlier, less sophisticated developmental stages, to gistful, spontaneous abstraction of relationship themes. Hence, patients are stimulated to think more as adults and less like prepubertal or early adolescent subjects. More specifically, CET strives to achieve 4 major goals. First and foremost, CET attempts to facilitate the attainment of social cognitive milestones that are appropriate for healthy adults. Among these milestones are the attainment of a 'gistfulness' in social exchange, effortful and active processing of social content, cognitive flexibility, a tolerance for ambiguity and uncertainty, and a personal comfort with abstraction. The second aim is to incite patients to display appropriate behavior in social contexts, which requires proper appraisal of the context as well as the ability to take another person's perspective. The third goal is to create a personally relevant understanding of schizophrenia by providing patients with psychoeducation. Patients may be more inclined to actively participate in planning and maintaining a treatment strategy that is specifically designed to meet their own cognitive difficulties, strengths and rehabilitation goals. Lastly, CET also addresses neuropsychological impairment, but in a more interactive process rather than with formal didactic exercises.

Therapy is conducted in small groups comprising 6–8 patients. Neurocognitive deficits are addressed by administering approximately 75 h of computer-based training that uses progressive exercises from the attention software of Ben-Yishay et al. [43] and the memory and problem-solving software of Bracy [45]. Computer sessions are conducted in pairs of patients with the therapist providing oversight. The patients take turns using the computer software programs and assist each other by providing strategies and offering encouragement. In addition, they receive approximately 56 sessions of social cognitive group exercises (1.5 h per week), containing activities such as categorization exercises, formation of gistful, condensed messages, solving real-life social dilemmas, abstraction of themes from the editorial pages of *USA Today*, appraisal of affect and social contexts, initiating and maintaining conversations, playwriting and the center stage exercises (e.g. introducing oneself or a friend) adapted from the curriculum of Ben-Yishay et al. [43]. Sessions typically include a homework review, a psychoeducation topic, an exercise by a patient or pair, feedback from other patients and coaches and a new homework assignment based on the education topic.

CET Efficacy Studies

Several studies have examined the effectiveness of CET. In a 2-year randomized controlled trial comprising 121 chronic schizophrenia and schizoaffective patients [46], CET was compared with enriched supportive therapy (EST) that incorporates components of personal therapy with its main focus on stress reduction strategies and psychoeducation (described elsewhere [47, 48]). All patients were in an outpatient setting, symptomatically stable and non-substance-abusing but showed cognitive disabilities. Neuropsychological and behavioral assessments were administered at baseline, as well as at 12 and 24 months and comprised the following measures: processing speed, neurocognition, cognitive style, social cognition, social adjustment and symptoms. Analysis of covariance as well as linear trend analysis was performed. The results indicated that at 12 months significant improvements were found for patients receiving CET compared to the group receiving EST for the neurocognition and processing speed composites and marginal effects emerged for the behavioral domains of cognitive style, social cognition and social adjustment. As was expected, no effect was observed on symptoms. By 24 months, recipients of CET not only continued to show enhanced cognition but also had significantly improved in all the behavioral domains with ES exceeding 1 SD except for symptoms. Patients receiving EST also improved on many composites after 2 years, surprisingly in particular on neurocognition. However, processing speed was unaffected by EST. The authors concluded that cognitive disabilities do not have to be persistent but can be ameliorated through adequate cognitive remediation. Moreover, these results suggest that improvement in functional outcome may be more likely achieved after longer periods of cognitive remediation.

A subsequent follow-up study [49] including 106 of the initial 121 patients who had received treatment favored CET over EST and revealed that 1 year after treatment end, recipients of CET maintained treatment gains in almost all the domains of cognition and behavior except for neurocognition. Although the neurocognition composite did not reach significance, the CET group did not deteriorate after the treatment had been ended, but rather neurocognition continued to improve in EST participants despite the absence of training. As in the previous studies, no effects were found for symptoms. In summary, CET constitutes an effective treatment with lasting effects for enhancing cognition in schizophrenia rehabilitation.

A further study conducted by Eack et al. [50] examined effects of CET on social cognition in early-course schizophrenia (n = 28) or schizoaffective disorder (n = 10), compared to previous studies where chronic schizophrenia patients had been examined. In order to meet the eligibility criteria, patients had to have received their diagnosis within the past 8 years. The average age was between 17 and 43 years, and the average length of illness was 3.75 years. The patients were randomly assigned to CET (n = 18) or EST (n = 20) and assessed at baseline and after a treatment phase of 1 year with the Mayer-Salovey-Caruso Emotional Intelligence Test [51], an objective, performance-based measure of emotional intelligence. The results showed large differential improvement on the overall emotional intelligence quotient for recipients of CET compared to participants of EST. The patients from the CET group even approached the average emotional intelligence quotient of healthy subjects. Furthermore, the participants of CET also improved significantly more than the recipients of the EST group in specific areas of emotional intelligence, such as in their ability to understand and manage emotions, and their capability to use emotions to facilitate thinking and decision making. Although a trend that CET compared to EST recipients' ability to accurately perceive emotions improved was observed, these findings did not emerge to be significant. These findings provide preliminary support for positive effects of CET on social cognition in early-course schizophrenia patients. Long-term effects of improved social cognition, specifically emotional intelligence, on functional outcome and social adjustment will be investigated in an ongoing, 2-year clinical trial [52].

Neurocognitive Enhancement Therapy (NET)

The NET is a comprehensive approach to cognitive remediation developed by Bell et al. [9, 53] with particular focus on work rehabilitation. NET is based upon models of neuroplasticity that highlight the need for intense and repetitive practice in order to target neurocognitive impairments. The program consists of 3 main components: computer-based cognitive training, a social information-processing group and a work feedback group. Cognitive exercises are based on a modified version of the multimedia CogReHab software that was originally designed for individuals with traumatic brain injury and other neurological impairments [54]. The repeated training sessions target cognitive functions such as attention, memory as well as executive function and take place 2–3 times per week, up to 5 h each week for 26 weeks. The tasks are initially designed to be relatively simple in order to allow patients to accomplish them. The level of difficulty hierarchically increases as soon as the participants attain 90% accuracy at a given degree of complexity. The patients are usually paid for doing cognitive exercises at USD 3.40 per hour with increasing bonus pay for reaching a maximum of 5 h of cognitive training. The group session for social information processing takes place weekly and resembles an exercise from the traumatic brain injury program of Ben-Yishay et al. [43]. One patient prepares an oral presentation with staff assistance and then introduces it to the group. Group members are required to ask questions and provide specific feedback. Over the 6 months, 3 topics are given in the following order: 'my job', 'a day at work' and 'what I've learned'. The third component addresses work feedback that includes ratings of job-related attention, memory and executive function and is provided biweekly by using the Cognitive Functional Assessment Scale. In addition, based on these feedbacks, patients are encouraged to develop new goals.

NET Efficacy Studies

A number of studies have evaluated the effectiveness of NET. In a trial comprising 65 patients with schizophrenia or schizoaffective disorder, participants were randomly assigned to NET plus work therapy (WT) or WT alone [9]. Both groups performed poorly on neuropsychological testing. After 5 months, greater improvements of executive function, working memory and affect recognition were found for patients receiving NET + WT.

A further study including 145 outpatients, either diagnosed as having schizophrenia or schizoaffective disorder, received 6 months of NET + WT or WT alone [55]. The results indicated that patients from the NET + WT condition worked more hours and earned more money than those from the WT group. During follow-up, patients who benefited from NET + WT worked the most hours and were engaged in more competitive wage employment.

In a study examining 152 patients with schizophrenia or schizoaffective disorder, performance on computerized training tasks as well as pre-post neuropsychological tests were measured after the patients had received either NET + WT or WT alone [56]. Prior to enrollment the patients had been divided into the 3 subgroups 'preserved intelligence', 'compromised intelligence' and 'deteriorated intelligence' based on their premorbid and morbid deficits. In general, the results revealed greater improvements for patients who had received NET + WT compared to those who had only received WT, but differences emerged for the different intellectual groups. In the compromised intelligence group, the ones from the NET + WT condition showed significantly more task normalization than the patients from the WT. In the preserved and the deteriorated intellectual groups, no such difference occurred. Contrariwise, subjects from the preserved and the deteriorated groups who had received NET + WT showed greater improvement in the neuropsychological test performance, which was not the case for the compromised group.

In a further study [57], 62 outpatients with a diagnosis of schizophrenia or schizo-affective disorder either participated in NET and a vocational program (VOC) or VOC only. The VOC included individual placement and support as well as transitional funding. After 1 year of treatment, participants receiving NET + VOC had significantly greater improvements on measures of executive function and working memory than those in the VOC only condition.

In a study comprising 72 outpatients with a schizophrenia diagnosis or schizoaffective disorder received NET + VOC or only VOC over a 12-month-period [58]. When the patients were divided into higher and lower community functioning, at a 12-months follow-up, only 11% of the patients with poor community function who had received VOC only became competitively employed as opposed to 60% of the NET + VOC patients with poor community function. Moreover, NET + VOC patients with poor community functioning worked twice as many hours as those who had received VOC only. Interestingly, over 60% of the higher community function patients achieved competitive employment regardless of whether they had received NET + VOC or VOC only. In addition, no difference in total hours worked was found in this group.

In conclusion, the findings support the efficacy of NET in enhancing cognitive functions and work outcomes. NET seems to be particularly beneficial for patients with poor community functioning.

Neuropsychological Educational Approach to Cognitive Remediation (NEAR)

The comprehensive, evidence-based, manualized NEAR developed by Medalia et al. [8] constitutes a synthesis of knowledge derived from educational psychology, behavior and learning theories, rehabilitation psychology and neuropsychology. NEAR postulates that cognitive remediation is in its essence a learning activity, wherefore educational principles, which promote intrinsic motivation and task engagement, are taken into account. This is of particular importance, as psychiatric illness like schizophrenia is not only accompanied by cognitive impairment but also by decreased motivation, avolition and apathy [59]. Patients are encouraged to reflect on their personal learning styles as many of them have encountered repeated failure in learning situations during adolescence due to their cognitive and social deficits. Together with the lack of motivation stemming from the illness itself, a negative attitude toward learning and cognitive activity is a frequent byproduct of these repeated experiences of failure. In order to promote a positive learning experience that elicits an intrinsic motivation to learn and use their cognitive skills, NEAR exercises are designed to be highly engaging, enjoyable and rewarding in and of themselves. The tasks are therefore presented in a contextualized, personalized, multisensory manner that also allows the learner to exert a certain level of control over nonessential aspects [60]. Independence, self-efficacy and persistence on learning tasks are fostered. Unlike other cognitive remediation methods, NEAR generally favors a top-down approach to remediation where tasks incorporate several skills simultaneously [61, 62].

Training is usually conducted 2–3 days a week in 45-min to 1-hour sessions with a group of up to 10 patients who each work at their own pace on tasks chosen to address their particular needs. Because the groups have rolling admission, there are opportunities for peer leadership as the more experienced participants lend their expertise to the newly enrolled members. Usually, patients perform computer-based cognitive tasks in 2 of 3 sessions and then in a third session attend a group meeting where social skills are practiced and the real-world relevance of the individually performed exercises is discussed. The tasks are taken from commercially available educational software that not only addresses various neuropsychological functions but is also designed to be engaging, enjoyable and intrinsically motivating. Clinicians who are in charge of group leadership are required to go through manualized training, practice and supervision of cognitive remediation and instructional techniques before being qualified to run a group [8]. For further information see chapter 5.1.

NEAR Efficacy Studies

A mixture of randomized controlled trials and community-based outcome studies have been used to examine whether NEAR is effective in the laboratory and in daily practice. The outcome measures typically include cognitive functioning and measures of real-world functioning such as treatment compliance, independent living skills, psychosocial functioning, psychiatric status, and educational and occupational advancement. Evidence that NEAR has a positive impact on cognitive functioning comes from a multisite randomized waiting list control trial of NEAR that was conducted with 40 participants with a diagnosis of schizophrenia or schizoaffective disorder who were between the ages of 17 and 50 [63]. The immediate treatment group received 20–30 sessions of NEAR over 15 weeks, while the waiting list group waited 15 weeks before starting their 20–30 sessions of NEAR. Both groups received standard TAU. Following treatment, significant improvements were found in the areas of attention, processing speed, executive functioning, and delayed verbal and visual memory. These gains were sustained 4 months after the treatment had ended.

Other randomized controlled trials with acute and chronic inpatients found that patients who received 6–10 sessions of NEAR exercises made significantly more improvement on verbal problem solving and problem-solving skills for independent living than patients in the control group [64, 65]. Furthermore, the gains in problem solving for independent living were sustained 1 month after the treatment had ended

[60]. A community-based outcome study with 48 mixed diagnosis patients found that 26 sessions of NEAR led to improvements in processing speed as used in a vocational task [66].

Several community-based outcome studies and 1 randomized controlled trial examined the impact of NEAR on measures of psychosocial functioning. The multisite randomized waiting list control trial conducted by Reblado-Hodge et al. [63] found that participants exposed to 20–30 sessions of NEAR in 15 weeks duration made significant improvements on the Social and Occupational Functioning Assessment Scale and sustained these gains 4 months after the treatment had ended [67]. One community-based outcome study [68] reported that as compared to mixed diagnosis outpatients who do not receive NEAR, those enrolled in a NEAR program become more engaged and productive in overall psychiatric treatment as measured by attendance at program, achievement of treatment goals and rates of hospitalization. Other community-based outcomes studies found that mixed diagnosis clients attending NEAR showedsignificantly improved work-related behaviors, and a 75% rate of discharge to educational and occupational placements [66, 69]. Taken together, these studies indicate that participation in NEAR impacts not only cognitive skills but psychosocial functioning as well.

Discussion

Altogether, the results for combined treatment approaches are encouraging and indicate improvements not only in proximal cognitive performance but also in the more distal areas of psychosocial functioning and psychopathology [27, 28]. Participation in adjunctive rehabilitation programs appears to have an advantage over programs with cognitive remediation alone [see [26] and is of great value for the recovery process in conjunction with medication, stationary and day care interventions. Therefore, it would be highly desirable to incorporate combined treatment approaches into standard care for schizophrenia patients. Despite differences in theoretical background and conceptualization of the combined approaches outlined above, patients were able to benefit from all of them, and, accordingly there seems to be no single best one. Rather, the choice of treatment should be based on individual needs and characteristics of the patients, carried out through behavior and problem analysis.

To facilitate the dissemination of cognitive remediation in clinical settings, further research is needed to clarify such issues as optimal treatment intensity, duration of treatment, group size, and best fit between treatment approach and patient population. Although no guidelines exist yet, it has been pointed out in the literature that more rather than fewer treatment sessions are better [70]. In addition, despite first indications that beneficial effects remain present after 1- or 2-year follow-ups, in order to maintain improvements in neurocognition and social cognition over a longer period of time, booster sessions may be necessary after treatment end. A further unanswered question concerns the significance of group versus individual settings in treatment. Previous research and clinical experience have shown that the group setting constitutes a highly effective treatment form for schizophrenia patients [2] as particularly social cognition and social competence may be activated automatically and can be practiced in a protected environment. Requirements for successful group treatments seem to be optimal structuring of the group, training of the therapists (i.e. they should be proficient in basic treatment techniques and create an atmosphere of acceptance, valuation as well as support), building group cohesion, promote intrinsic motivation and optimal relational shaping (i.e. regulation of proximity and distance) [also see 20]. Nevertheless, to date, it remains unclear whether the group setting per se brings upon improvement (indirect effect) or if the structured neurocognition-enhancing or social skill exercises produce the main advantage (direct effect). Future research should shed more light on group therapy, group processes and effectiveness mechanisms of group treatments. Another interesting question regards the relation between social cognition and social skills. Should social cognition and social skills be seen as more independent therapy entities or how do they interact? For example, positive experiences may alter paranoid attributions, schemas or social perception. Contrariwise, modified attributions may lead to more adequate social behavior. An existing connection would have direct treatment implications. Lastly, mediating and moderating factors should be taken into account in order to develop more individualized treatments. Interventions should ideally be designed according to patients' cognitive profile, length and phase of illness. Previous research [71] has shown that intellectually compromised patients are more likely to benefit from compensatory inventions, whereas those with fewer cognitive deficits may profit more from cognition-enhancing programs. Moreover, patients with broad cognitive deficits or a long duration of illness may need an extended course of treatment. Ultimately, therapies which customize the instructional techniques to the patient's personal recovery needs are most likely to be consistent with better outcomes, and the treatments which are able to address both neurocognitive and social cognitive deficits provide a broad base from which to build psychiatric recovery.

References

1 Kurtz MM, Mueser KT: Social skills training for schizophrenia: a meta-analysis of controlled research. J Consult Clin Psychol 2008;76:491–504.
2 Roder V, Mueller DR, Brenner HD, Spaulding WD: Integrated Psychological Therapy for Schizophrenia Patients (IPT). Göttingen, Hogrefe, in press.
3 Delahunty A, Morice R: A Training Programme for the Remediation of Cognitive Deficits in Schizophrenia. Albury, Department of Health of Australia, 1993.
4 Wykes T, Reeder C, Corner J, Williams C, Everitt B: The effects of neurocognitive remediation on executive processing in patients with schizophrenia. Schizophr Bull 1999;25:291–307.
5 Wykes T, Reeder C, Williams C, Corner J, Rice C, Everitt B: Are the effects of cognitive remediation therapy (CRT) durable? Results from an exploratory trial in schizophrenia. Schizophr Res 2003;61:163–174.

6   Delahunty A, Reeder C, Wykes T, Morice R, Newton E: Revised Cognitive Remediation Therapy Manual. London, Institute of Psychiatry, 2002.

7   Roder V, Lächler M, Müller DR: Integrated Neurocognitive Therapy for Schizophrenia Patients (INT). Swiss National Foundation, Grant No 3200 B0–108133.

8   Medalia A, Revheim N, Herlands T: Cognitive Remediation for Psychological Disorders. Therapist Guide. New York, Oxford University Press, 2009.

9   Bell M, Bryson G, Greig T, Corcoran C, Wexler BE: Neurocognitive enhancement therapy with work therapy: effects on neuropsychological test performance. Arch Gen Psychiatry 2001;58:763–768.

10 Andreasen NC, Carpenter WT, Kane JM, Lasser RA, Marder SR, Weinberger DR: Remission in schizophrenia: proposed criteria and rationale for consensus. Am J Psychiatry 2005;162:441–449.

11 Green MF, Nuechterlein KH: Should schizophrenia be treated as a neurocognitive disorder? Schizophr Bull 1999;25:309–318.

12 Vauth R, Rusch N, Wirtz M, Corrigan PW: Does social cognition influence the relation between neurocognitive deficits and vocational functioning in schizophrenia? Psychiatry Res 2004;128:155–165.

13 Brekke J, Kay DD, Lee KS, Green MF: Biosocial pathways to functional outcome in schizophrenia. Schizophr Res 2005;80:213–225.

14 Sergi MJ, Rassovsky Y, Nuechterlein KH, Green MF: Social perception as a mediator of the influence of early visual processing on functional status in schizophrenia. Am J Psychiatry 2006;163:448–454.

15 Sergi MJ, Green MF, Widmark C, Reist C, Erhart S, Braff DL, Kee KS, Marder SR, Mintz J: Social cognition and neurocognition: effects of risperidone, olanzapine, and haloperidol. Am J Psychiatry 2007;164:1585–1592.

16 Bell M, Tsang HWH, Greig TC, Bryson GJ: Neurocognition, social cognition, perceived social discomfort, and vocational outcomes in schizophrenia. Schizophr Bull 2009;35:738–747.

17 Aleman A, Agrawal N, Morgan KD, Davis AS: Insight in psychosis and neuropsychological function. Br J Psychiatry 2006;189:204–212.

18 Velligan DI, Robert SK, Gold JM: Cognitive rehabilitation for schizophrenia and the putative role of motivation and expectancies. Schizophr Bull 2006;32:474–485.

19 Medalia A, Lim R: Treatment of cognitive dysfunction in psychiatric disorders. J Psychiatr Pract 2004;10:17–25.

20 Medalia A, Richardson R: What predicts a good response to cognitive remediation interventions? Schizophr Bull 2005;31:942–953.

21 Resnick SG, Rosenheck RA, Lehmann AF: An exploratory analysis of correlates of recovery. Psychiatr Serv 2004;55:540–547.

22 Corrigan PW: Recovery of schizophrenia and the role of evidence-based psychological interventions. Expert Rev Neurother 2006;7:993–1004.

23 Kurtz MM, Moberg PJ, Gur RC, Gur RE: Approaches to cognitive remediation of neuropsychological deficits in schizophrenia: a review and meta-analysis. Neuropsychol Rev 2001;11:197–210.

24 Pilling S, Bebbington P, Kuipers E, Garety P, Geddes J, Martindale B, Orbach G, Morgan C: Psychological treatments in schizophrenia. II. Meta-analyses of randomized controlled trials of social skills training and cognitive remediation. Schizophr Bull 2002;32:783–791.

25 Krabbendam L, Aleman A: Cognitive rehabilitation in schizophrenia: a quantitative analysis of controlled studies. Psychopharmacology 2003;169:376–382.

26 Twamley EW, Jeste DV, Bellack AS: A review of cognitive training in schizophrenia. Schizophr Bull 2003;29:359–382.

27 Pfammatter M, Junghan UM, Brenner HD: Efficacy of psychological therapy in schizophrenia: conclusions from meta-analyses. Schizophr Bull 2006;32:64–80.

28 McGurk SR, Twamley EW, Sitzer DI, McHugo GJ, Mueser KT: A meta-analysis of cognitive remediation in schizophrenia. Am J Psychiatry 2007;164:1791–1802.

29 Wexler BE, Bell MD: Cognitive remediation and vocational rehabilitation for schizophrenia. Schizophr Bull 2005;31:931–941.

30 American Psychological Association Committee for the Advancement of Professional Practice Task Force on Serious Mental Illness and Severe Emotional Disturbance: Training grid outlining best practices for recovery and improved outcomes for people with serious mental illness. http://www.apa.org/practice/smi_grid-v2.pdf (accessed June 2009).

31 Brenner HD, Hodel B, Roder V, Corrigan P: Treatment of cognitive dysfunctions and behavioral deficits in schizophrenia: Integrated Psychological Therapy. Schizophr Bull 1992;18:21–26.

32 Roder V, Brenner HD, Kienzle N: Integriertes Psychologisches Therapieprogramm bei schizophren Erkrankten IPT, ed 6, rev. Weinheim, Beltz, 2008.

33 Roder V, Mueller DR, Mueser KT, Brenner HD: Integrated Psychological Therapy (IPT) for schizophrenia: is it effective? Schizophr Bull 2006;32:81–93.

34 Mueller DR, Roder V: Empirical evidence for group therapy addressing social perception in schizophrenia; in Teiford JB (ed): Social perception: 21st Century Issues and Challenges. New York, Nova Science Publishers, 2008, pp 51–80.

35 Pilling S, Bebbington P, Kuipers E, Garety P, Geddes J, Orbach G, Morgan C: Psychological treatments in schizophrenia. I. Meta-analyses of family intervention and cognitive behaviour therapy. Psychol Med 2002;32:763–782.

36 Green MF, Olivier B, Crawley JN, Penn DL, Silverstein S: Social cognition in schizophrenia: recommendations from the measurement and treatment research to improve cognition in schizophrenia new approaches conference. Schizophr Res 2005;31: 882–887.

37 Nuechterlein KH, Barch DM, Gold JM, Goldberg TE, Green MF, Heaton RK: Identification of separable cognitive factors in schizophrenia. Schizophr Res 2004;72:29–39.

38 Roder V, Mueller D: Integrated Neurocognitive Therapy (INT) for Schizophrenia Patients. Unpublished manual. Bern, University Hospital of Psychiatry, 2006.

39 Hogarty GE, Greenwald DP, Eack SM: Durability and mechanism of effects of cognitive enhancement therapy. Psychiatr Serv 2006;57:1751–1757.

40 Hogarty GE, Flesher S, Ulrich R, Carter M, Greenwald D, Pogue-Geile M, Kechavan M, Cooley S, Louise DiBarry A, Garrett A, Parepally H, Zoretich R: Cognitive enhancement therapy for schizophrenia: effects of a 2-year randomized trial on cognition and behavior. Arch Gen Psychiatry 2004; 61:866–876.

41 Hogarty GE, Flesher S: Practice principles of cognitive enhancement therapy for schizophrenia. Schizophr Bull 1999;25:693–708.

42 Hogarty GE, Flesher S: Developmental theory for a cognitive enhancement therapy of schizophrenia. Schizophr Bull 1999;25:677–692.

43 Ben-Yishay Y, Rattok J, Lakin P, Piasetsky E, Ross B, Silver S, Zide E, Ezrachi O: Neuropsychological rehabilitation: quest for a holistic approach. Semin Neurol 1985;5:252–259.

44 Brainerd CJ, Reyna VF: Gist is the grist: fuzzy trace theory and the new intuitionism. Dev Rev 1990;10: 3–47.

45 Bracy O: CET Computer-assisted training exercises. Indianapolis, Neuroscience Center of Indianapolis, 2003. www.Neuroscience.cnter.com/pss/psscogrehab/index.htm.

46 Hogarty GE, Flesher S, Ulrich R, Carter M, Greenwald D, Pogue-Geile M, Kechavan M, Cooley S, DiBarry AL, Garrett A, Parepally H, Zoretich R: Cognitive enhancement therapy for schizophrenia: effects of a 2-year randomized trial on cognition and behavior. Arch Gen Psychiatry 2004;61:866–876.

47 Hogarty GE, Greenwald D, Ulrich RF, Kornblith SJ, DiBarry AL, Cooley S, Carter M, Flesher S: Three-year trials of personal therapy among schizophrenic patients living within or independent of family. II. Effects on adjustment of patients. Am J Psychiatry 1997;154:1514–1524.

48 Hogarty GE: Personal Therapy for Schizophrenia and Related Disorders. A Guide to Individualized Treatment. New York, Guilford Press, 2002.

49 Hogarty GE, Greenwald DP, Eack SM: Durability and mechanism of effects of cognitive enhancement therapy. Psychiatr Serv 2006;57:1751–1757.

50 Eack SM, Hogarty GE, Greenwald DP, Hogarty SS, Keshavan MS: Cognitive enhancement therapy improves emotional intelligence in early course schizophrenia: preliminary effects. Schizophr Res 2007;89:308–311.

51 Mayer JD, Salovey P, Caruso DR, Sitarenios G: Measuring emotional intelligence with the MSCEIT V2.0. Emotion 2003;3:97–105.

52 Keshavan M: Rehabilitation, brain function and early schizophrenia. NIMH Grant MH60902, 2005.

53 Bell M, Zito W, Greig T, Wexler BE: Neurocognitive enhancement therapy and competitive employment in schizophrenia: effects on clients with poor community functioning. Am J Psychiatr Rehabil 2008; 11:109–122.

54 Bracy O: CogRehab Software. Indianapolis, Psychological Software Services, 1995.

55 Wexler BE, Bell MD: Cognitive remediation and vocational rehabilitation for schizophrenia. Schizophr Bull 2005;31:931–941.

56 Fiszdon JM, Choi J, Bryson GJ, Bell MD: Impact of intellectual status on response to cognitive task training in patients with schizophrenia. Schizophr Res 2006;87:261–269.

57 Greig TC, Zito W, Wexler BE, Fiszon J, Bell MD: Improved cognitive function in schizophrenia after one year of cognitive training and vocational services. Schizophr Res 2007;96:156–161.

58 Bell MD, Zito W, Greig T, Wexler BE: Neurocognitive enhancement therapy with vocational services: work outcomes at two-year follow-up. Schizophr Res 2008;105:18–29.

59 Medalia A, Freilich B: The neuropsychological educational approach to cognitive remediation (NEAR) model: practice principles and outcome studies. Am J Psychiatr Rehabil 2008;11:123–143.

60 Medalia A, Revheim N, Casey M: Remediation of problem-solving skills in schizophrenia: evidence of a persistent effect. Schizophr Res 2002;57:165–171.

61 Medalia A, Richardson R: What predicts a good response to cognitive remediation interventions? Schizophr Bull 2005;31:942–953.

62 Schwalbe E, Medalia A: Cognitive dysfunction and competency restoration: using cognitive remediation to help restore the unrestorable. J Am Acad Psychiatry Law 2007;35:518–525.

63 Redoblado-Hodge MA, Siciliano D, Withey P, Moss B, Moore G, Judd G, Shores EA, Harris A: A randomized controlled trial of cognitive remediation in schizophrenia. Schizophr Bull 2008, Epub ahead of print.

64 Medalia A, Revheim N, Casey M: The remediation of problem-solving skills in schizophrenia. Schizophr Bull 2001;27:259–267.

65 Medalia A, Dorn H, Watras-Gans S: Treating problem-solving deficits on an acute care psychiatric inpatient unit. Psychiatry Res 2000;97:79–88.

66 Choi J, Medalia A: Factors associated with a positive response to cognitive remediation in a community psychiatric sample. Psychiatr Serv 2005;56:602–604.

67 Goldman NH, Skodol AE, Lave TR: Revising axis V for DSM-IV; a review of measures of social functioning. Am J Psychiatry 1992;49:1148–1156.

68 Revheim N, Kamnitzer D, Casey M, Medalia A: Implementation of a cognitive rehabilitation program in an IPRT setting. Psychiatr Rehabil Skills 2001;5:403–425.

69 Medalia A, Herlands T, Baginsky C: Rehab rounds: cognitive remediation in the supportive housing setting. Psychiatr Serv 2003;54:1219–1120.

70 Heydebrand G: Issues in rehabilitation of cognitive deficits in schizophrenia: a critical review. Curr Psychiatry Rev 2007;3:186–195.

71 Mao-Sheng R, Eric Yu-Hai C: Cognitive enhancement therapy for schizophrenia. Lancet 2004;364: 2163–2165.

Prof. Volker Roder
University Hospital of Psychiatry
Bolligenstrasse 111
CH–3000 Bern 60 (Switzerland)
Tel. +41 31 930 99 07, Fax +41 31 930 99 88, E-Mail roder@sunrise.ch

Roder V, Medalia A (eds): Neurocognition and Social Cognition in Schizophrenia Patients. Basic Concepts and Treatment. Key Issues Ment Health. Basel, Karger, 2010, vol 177, pp 104–117

5.1

An Overview of the Neuropsychological and Educational Approach to Remediation

Alice Medalia · Elisa Mambrino

Department of Psychiatry, Columbia University College of Physicians and Surgeons, New York, N.Y., USA

Abstract

The Neuropsychological Educational Approach to Remediation (NEAR) is a treatment framework designed specifically to provide psychiatric patients across the diagnostic spectrum with integrated remediation in cognition and social role functioning. This chapter discusses NEAR's theoretical underpinnings, basic program structure and techniques. Cognitive deficits that accompany severe and persistent mental illness impinge upon functional outcome and present patients of all ages with a variety of cognitive, social and emotional challenges during neuropsychiatric rehabilitation and recovery. The complexity of patient need is reflected in NEAR's multidisciplinary stance, which includes 2 core components, individualized cognitive training and a bridging group. These components work hand in hand using techniques that enhance intrinsic motivation to learn, cognition and functional outcome.
Copyright © 2010 S. Karger AG, Basel

The Neuropsychological Educational Approach to Remediation (NEAR) is one of a number of evidence-based approaches to cognitive remediation, and it was designed specifically for psychiatric patients. It provides a practical framework for the delivery of treatment across settings, including hospital- and community-based programs. With roots in neuropsychology, rehabilitation psychology, educational psychology, self-determination theory and client-centered therapy, NEAR was designed for a diagnostic spectrum of patients who range in age from adolescent to geriatric. In both theoretical principle and corresponding practical application, NEAR's integrated approach places a premium not only on improving cognitive skills but also mediating the remediation process by enhancing the patient's related sense of competency, engaging a patient's intrinsic motivation and improving psychosocial functioning at home, at school, at work and in the community.

To achieve these ends, NEAR provides a multimodal treatment approach using individualized cognitive remediation accompanied by a group component. The patients work in a group on their own computer to complete a customized program of commercially available computer exercises designed to improve the neurocognitive functions identified as sufficient to hamper the patient's functional outcome. The specially trained NEAR clinician monitors activities to assure that the patient develops a sense of competence and confidence necessary to acquire and apply cognitive skills specially targeted in remediation. Group treatment then 'bridges' the gap between cognitive remediation skills learned in isolation and provides patients with practice in applying cognitive skills in everyday contexts. From design to implementation, NEAR aims to provide a positive learning experience to each and every patient, improve independent learning skills and nurture a positive attitude about learning. By promoting awareness about learning style as well as individual learning strengths and weaknesses, the NEAR clinician encourages patients to take as active a role as possible in optimizing their cognitive functioning, practicing social role skills and discussing how the individualized cognitive exercises they are working on relate to real-world activities and challenges.

In order to better understand the basis of NEAR's multidisciplinary approach to cognitive remediation, the following section provides a discussion of the theories that support the treatment framework.

Theories That Inform NEAR

Neuropsychology

For patients with severe and persistent mental illness, psychiatric interventions do not significantly enhance cognitive functioning. As a result, cognitive deficits remain entrenched even after an individual has been psychiatrically stabilized. Chronic neurocognitive impairment is a significant predictor of social and vocational outcomes because it has a negative influence on so many fundamental aspects of daily living, including treatment response, compliance with psychiatric care, schooling, employment, social relationships, living arrangements and community functioning [1].

To cure the chronic cognitive impairments that accompany schizophrenia, the field of psychiatry turned to neuropsychology to create a behavioral treatment designed specifically to target cognitive impairments associated with functional psychosocial decline. Neuropsychology's emphasis on brain-behavior relationships utilized neurophysiology and neuroanatomy to conceptualize the nature of cognitive deficits in need of remediation. Neuropsychology also provided a bottom-up or traditionally hierarchical view of cognitive processes, in which attention is regarded as the most basic process that makes possible much more complex, executive problem solving.

NEAR appreciates the value of a hierarchical view of cognition and uses that perspective as one way to evaluate activities. However, NEAR departs from the more traditional, bottomup neuropsychological approach to cognitive remediation by also providing training on tasks that incorporate several skills at once in a contextualized format. This approach not only elicits several types of response in concert, thus simulating real-life cognitive tasks, but also allows for more flexibility in designing tasks that are engaging enough to keep the patient motivated to participate in treatment.

NEAR also relies on basic neuropsychological principles to understand the way patients approach cognitive tasks. This takes the process approach to neuropsychological assessment initially advocated by Edith Kaplan [2] and applies it to the treatment realm. The NEAR clinician is taught to place less emphasis on the numeric indices of advancement on a task and more on how the patient approached the task. By using a process approach, performance on cognitive training tasks becomes a window onto the neuropsychological bases for daily dysfunction. For example, a patient may fail at sorting items into a Venn diagram and obtain a low score for any single reason or a combination of reasons: failure to form sets (executive dysfunction), failure to remember the sorting principles (working memory) or failure to complete the task in time (processing speed). If the clinician focused importance on just the score alone, he/she would miss valuable information about the nature of the patient's cognitive dysfunction. On the other hand, a process approach to analyzing the patient's performance on a given cognitive task allows the clinician to analyze underlying cognitive processing problems, design a treatment plan to address the relevant cognitive deficits as well as refine and update the treatment over time as changes in a patient's neuropsychiatric recovery and or developmental level unfold.

To design cognitive remediation for psychiatric patients, neuropsychologists took inspiration from colleagues who treated brain-injured patients [3, 4]. In addition to providing a model for cognitive training tasks, there was much to learn from the general models of treatment that were used. Individuals who experienced traumatic brain injury typically showed some progress in structured clinic-based tasks. However, their performance in the real world did not readily or automatically improve in kind because the patients had difficulty generalizing what they learned to cognitively complex psychosocial tasks performed in a real-world environment [5].

NEAR was particularly inspired by the holistic or global approach to cognitive remediation advocated by Ben Yishay and Diller [3]. Their 'substitutive' or 'compensatory' approach emphasizes the importance of problem solving, the development and transfer of compensatory strategies, and the patient's awareness of his or her relative select cognitive strengths and weaknesses. An emphasis on metacognition and executive control exercises helps the patient deconstruct tasks and self-monitor their own problem solving. Ben Yishay and Diller argued that a holistic or integrative approach is vital to remediation, and therefore it is necessary to therapeutically address issues of awareness, self-concept and self-efficacy in addition to the neurocognitive skills.

Rehabilitation Psychology

Rehabilitation psychology is related to neuropsychology but is a separate specialty area of practice that appreciates the complex interaction of cognitive, emotional and environmental variables in the recovery process [4, 6]. By addressing recovery as a process, as opposed to just targeting cognitive issues, rehabilitation psychology emphasizes the social emotional as well as the cognitive needs of the patient. Diller [7] termed this an 'ecological' approach. It considers the interrelationship between and among factors related to the patient's recovery and the social-emotional environment in which recovery takes place.

NEAR is intended to be used within the context of a rehabilitation program that offers patients training in the educational, vocational, social and independent living skills necessary for recovery and reintegration into society. Accordingly, the treatment framework focuses on cognition as it is used in social-emotional contexts.

Behavioral and Learning Theory

Behavior and learning theories provide us with an understanding of the process of learning. Drawing from the extensive literature in these fields, NEAR incorporates several concepts that have been found to promote learning and task engagement. For example, shaping, errorless learning and generalization are commonly used to facilitate learning. Shaping refers to the gradual changes in behavior in response to incremental, corrective reinforcement. Errorless learning [8] includes the careful titration of difficulty level so that the learner does not have to resort to trial-and-error learning. Generalization refers to the transfer of a learned skill or behavior to other situations besides the one where the training occurred, and it is another concept derived from learning theory which is critical to NEAR. Within the remediation exercises, target behaviors need to be paired with multiple cues, ideally in various contexts so that the behavior will be elicited in multiple settings. New learning is said to generalize when newly learned information or strategies are transferred and applied in a different context or learning domain.

Educational Psychology

Educational psychology has made significant contributions to an understanding of the conditions under which optimal learning can take place and some of the best strategies for effective instruction. Whereas it was once thought that learning is directly correlated with intellectual ability, educational psychology has refocused the field on the other factors that also have an impact on learning, namely instructional techniques and motivation to learn [9–11].

Research with students has shown that they learn the most, learn the fastest and retain knowledge the longest when they are excited and motivated for the pleasure of learning, exploring, seeking challenge and testing their abilities [12–14]. Without apparent need for external or extrinsic rewards, persuasion or pressure, intrinsically motivated individuals find performance of the task rewarding in and of itself. This type of excitement about learning is called intrinsic motivation. Research has shown that when people are pressured through the use of external incentives, deadlines and authoritarian commentary, they are less likely to be intrinsically motivated. As a result, extrinsically motivated people are less likely to learn as much or perform to the best of their ability [15].

One way to promote intrinsic motivation and task engagement is to use tasks that are contextualized, personalized and allow for learner control [12]. Contextualization means that rather than presenting material in the abstract, information is instead put in a context whereby the practical utility and link to everyday life activities are obvious to the patient. Personalization refers to the tailoring of a learning activity to coincide with topics of high interest value for the patient. Learner control can be gained by offering the patient the opportunity to choose from among a forced-choice menu of activities. For example, people exert control over a learning situation when they choose auditory over visual presentation, or when they determine the difficulty level.

Since apathy, anhedonia and avolition are frequent symptoms in the severely mentally ill and these motivational problems can compromise engagement in treatment, NEAR uses teaching techniques with psychiatric patients that will increase their sense of intrinsic motivation and engagement with cognitive remediation. Besides improved compliance with treatment recommendations [16], intrinsic motivation is also associated with other benefits, including increased levels of self-determination, autonomy and sense of well-being [17].

Self-Determination Theory

Self-determination theory is an approach to personality and motivation that examines how the interplay of social-contextual conditions and innate psychological needs fosters constructive development, well-being, happiness and optimal functioning [17]. Self-determination refers to the factors that influence the development of the self. According to this theory, optimal development of the self occurs when people are intrinsically motivated and self-regulating and when their basic psychological needs are met. Basic psychological needs are identified as competence, autonomy and relatedness. When these are met, people become more intrinsically motivated and they learn more efficiently.

NEAR has identified instructional techniques to enhance opportunities to meet the basic needs for competency, autonomy and relatedness so that patients will be more intrinsically motivated to improve cognitive functioning. The group format, use of peer leaders and availability of choices within the exercises and curriculum are examples of ways that NEAR fosters self-determination and intrinsic motivation to learn.

Client-Centered Therapy of Carl Rogers

Carl Rogers [18] is best known for his development of client-centered therapy and counseling techniques, but he also was very interested in the relationship between educator and student. He referred to the teacher as a facilitator, reflecting a belief that enactive learning is more effective than direct teaching. In this spirit, NEAR clinicians are encouraged to view themselves as facilitators who create an environment for engagement in the learning process, value the patient's feelings, learning style and opinions, and conduct NEAR groups in a caring, nonauthoritative way that will facilitate learning.

Another important principle of client-centered therapy is that the clinician's ability to feel and convey genuineness, acceptance and empathy are 'core conditions' for facilitating learning [18]. Rogers also wrote about the importance of teachers and clinicians as facilitators who are able to understand a student's reactions to the learning process without judging, a process he called empathetic understanding. In NEAR, the clinician uses this understanding to better guide the learning process, enhance the dialogue with the patient about metacognition and explore the patient's unique approach to learning.

NEAR's Basic Program Structure

The NEAR program has two principal treatment modalities, and they work hand in hand: individualized cognitive training and a supportive bridging group. Taken together, the cognitive training and the bridging group are designed to enhance motivation and facilitate the learning and application of remediated cognitive skills. Improvements in basic cognitive skills associated with attention, concentration, memory and verbal skills enhance functioning in situations encountered in real-life settings at home, at school and at work.

Typically, one clinician works with three to nine patients who assemble twice a week for a total of two hours of computer exercises and once a week for 45 minutes of bridging group exercises. Twice weekly cognitive training in the form of individualized computer-based exercises allows patients to hone their skills using neuroscience and educational software chosen for content and level of difficulty, based on the results of each participant's baseline screening or test data. The individualized program of cognitive training takes a process approach to learning, and it is constantly evaluated and modified to assure that the program of exercises reflects the demonstrated cognitive and motivational needs of the patient, as they are manifest in their daily progress toward their recovery goals.

For all patients, weekly bridging group therapy sessions accompany the individualized cognitive training and are an indispensible part of the NEAR architecture. Generalization or the transfer of skills from one domain of learning to a broader context is an automatic process in healthy individuals but requires specific, targeted interventions in individuals with cognitive deficits. As its name suggests, the bridging group provides that support and practice in cognitive skills. Learning transfer is addressed across group tasks, by putting cognitive skills into action in group role playing, group problem solving and direct group instruction.

Rolling admission to the NEAR program assures a steady enrollment of patients and allows for a balance of advanced and novice participants to contribute to a productive group learning process. In cognitive remediation, the mix of experienced and novice learners reminds patients that learning is an ongoing process. Even as patients work alone at computer exercises, they know there are others in the room who are also working toward getting better and re-entering society at the degree that individual circumstances permit. For patients with severe and persistent mental illness, tolerating the mere presence of others may be an important first step in decreasing social isolation. In the bridging group, the range of experienced and novice learners provides opportunities for participants to discuss learning at various levels. This promotes cohesion among patients, who share excitement about the practical value of learning and their own experiences about the learning process itself as well as provide some solace or practical tips to one another when learning is difficult.

The following sections illustrate how each of NEAR's two components is designed to enhance both cognition and functional outcome in complementary ways.

Techniques to Enhance Cognition

Cognitive Training Groups

NEAR favors a customized approach to the delivery of cognitive remediation. Each patient is started on a program of cognitive exercises based on the results of an individual screening session which assesses both cognition and relevant psychosocial history. The computer-based training curriculum provides drill and practice on cognitive tasks, with activities that may concentrate on single or multiple cognitive domains. Computer-based training exercises target such areas of cognition as working memory, memory, logic and reasoning, attention, processing speed and problem solving.

The clinician carefully chooses from among a variety of computerized tasks that are engaging and that address each patient's cognitive strengths, weaknesses as well as functional needs. A 'Building Block' approach is used as a guide to session planning, with learning levels increasing in complexity along four dimensions: task utility value, task difficulty, cognitive load and task goal property. Task value relates the specific cognitive skill to a functional recovery goal (e.g., improve sustained attention to pass a math test). Task difficulty includes the number and intricacy of steps needed to complete the exercise. Cognitive load refers to the cognitive domains targeted in the activity and task goal property whether task completion involves working toward a highly proximal, well-defined goal or a more distal, vaguely defined goal. From basic to intermediate to advanced, this 'Building Block' approach gradually allows the participant to receive training in each cognitive skill necessary for higher-order executive functioning.

The clinician uses these four dimensions as criterion for targeting and remediating a particular cognitive skill at any given level of difficulty, whether it is beginning, intermediate or advanced. For each patient, customizing a program of cognitive remediation tasks to address a given cognitive skill requires the clinician to consider and address several factors at once to individualize the patient's program: the clinician must judge and select tasks based upon how they would best suit the patient's current cognitive skill level revealed in baseline testing (task difficulty, cognitive load) and address the patient's individual recovery goals (task utility value). Furthermore, the clinician considers whether the tasks have goal properties appropriate to the patient's cognitive and emotional capacity to work on proximal versus distal or well-defined versus vague goals. For example, a patient with low self-confidence and poor attention would be better suited to a task with proximal, well-defined goals. The individualized nature of the session plans helps prevent the frustration that can result from a one-size-fits-all program that may be too difficult or easy for any given patient or otherwise not address their specific cognitive profile. Individualizing a program of cognitive remediation increases the likelihood that a patient will be sufficiently but not overly challenged and receive sufficient learning support in a milieu that is conducive to enhancing motivation while promoting a positive sense of self.

The clinician introduces activities based upon the building block approach to session planning. Each building block is composed of sessions that introduce an assortment of computerized cognitive exercises rated along the above four dimensions. The actual software activities that are utilized change as software becomes obsolete or new activities are developed and placed on the market. Using a rubric developed to evaluate the appropriateness of software [19], clinicians are able to choose from a large array of cognitive activities that reflect the latest developments in the field of cognitive software exercises.

Building Block 1 introduces basic cognitive skills like attention and working memory, using tasks that have proximal goals, good face validity and low cognitive load. This format facilitates self-efficacy and task valuation, which in turn enhances motivation, decreases frustration and improves the likelihood that the participant will remain in the program and proceed to the next block of computer exercises. Patients

Table 1. Building Blocks to Cognitive Enhancement

Building Block 1: Basic skills	Task interest and attainment value are salient motivators for more impaired patients (e.g., 'I want to be like that patient who looks smart. He is working on a task that looks interesting to me'). The utility value is evident to higher functioning patients but must be taught to more impaired participants so they relate activity to functional goals (I want to improve my memory so I won't forget appointments). The task difficulty level is easy and emphasizes basic cognitive skills, e.g. selective attention or working memory. The cognitive load is low so that the patient does not juggle learning more than one skill at a time. The task goal properties are specific and proximal so that motivation is maximized
Building Block 2: Intermediate skills	The task utility value is emphasized (e.g., 'This skill will help me pay attention to take a test at school'); the interest value is also important. The task level of difficulty is intermediate, e.g., memory and concept formation. The cognitive load is intermediate in intensity. The goal properties of the task are increasingly more complex and distal
Building Block 3: Advanced skills	The task utility value takes precedence. The task level of difficulty is relatively advanced, e.g., complex problem solving. The cognitive load is relatively high and requires juggling more than one skill. The task goal properties are complex and distal

vary in the amount of time they require this basic level of training. For some, many sessions over a period of months are devoted to Building Block 1 exercises. For others, they may rapidly move to the next level in a matter of days. However, even those who move quickly to the next level may devote a small portion of their subsequent sessions to basic training exercises. Building Block 2 introduces intermediate cognitive skills like memory and concept formation (similarity and differences) using tasks that have slightly more distal goals, good face validity and a somewhat more complex cognitive load. Building Block 3 introduces complex cognitive skills like problem solving using tasks with even more distal goals (perhaps requiring multiple sessions to complete), good face validity and complex cognitive load. NEAR's Building Blocks are illustrated in table 1.

The building block approach provides a general rubric for designing a treatment plan in a clinical setting or a fixed program of activities for research settings where standardization of treatment is essential. In the clinic setting, the clinician uses the rubric to guide a staging of exercises, but there is more room for individualizing the protocol than in a research setting. Therefore, in a clinic setting it is not unusual to see patients doing exercises from two building blocks in any given session, even though across sessions they may generally spend more time on one block of exercises than another. Or, if patients are in the midst of a stressful time or relapse, they may benefit from returning to the previous block of exercises, to regain their focus and confidence. In the research setting, there are also ways to allow for this more fluid approach to treatment planning. For example, by building some 'free choice' time into each session, there is an opportunity for the patient to take an active role in customizing their plan of cognitive training. That may include a return to activities from a previous block of exercises.

NEAR clinicians are trained in motivational techniques to enrich the group environment. For example, giving patients more autonomy and decentralizing decision-making processes fosters patients' ability to take risks in learning new cognitive tasks. Patients are instrumental in setting their own functional goals and choosing from a forced-choice menu of cognitive remediation tasks that should facilitate goal attainment. When patients assemble in a room and sit down at computers to work individually on cognitive remediation tasks, the clinician works with them on a one-to-one basis, going around the room showing people new tasks, coaching those who are having difficulty and using a process approach to watch how engaged patients perform their tasks. While there are several patients assembled in a room at any given time, each participant works at his or her own pace on computerized cognitive remediation tasks selected to meet their recovery goals. If they so wish or prefer, two patients may work together if the clinician believes the arrangement would be beneficial to both of them. It is up to the clinician to monitor all aspects of the environment, to maximize learning, respect and reciprocity between and among patients.

Each participant is taught to monitor his or her own performance on paper in the form of tracking sheets. The clinician helps each patient maintain daily tracking sheets in a folder which provides a concrete and ongoing log of the patient's activities. Research has shown that people who are continually made self-aware of their performance and cognitive activity level seem to engage in a self-monitoring process that has been shown to improve the outcome in cognitive remediation [20, 21]. In an instance when the patient's tracking sheets indicate that progress is poor, this would be a signal to the clinician to intervene and adjust the patient's cognitive remediation program, using criteria from the four dimensions discussed above. Then, according to the process approach to analyzing the reasons for poor performance, the clinician may encourage the patient to work on a different activity. This flexibility in session planning insures that the remediation program can meet the patient's needs, which may change over time.

Bridging Groups

The bridging group is yet another layer of the NEAR model that is used to enhance cognition in ways that range from the concrete to the intangible. Small group discussions facilitate the transfer of skills by emphasizing and reinforcing the practical ways in which basic cognitive skills are used every day (e.g., how to use categorization techniques to organize a weekly schedule). The bridging group provides direct instruction on how to apply cognitive skills to real-world tasks and gives opportunities to practice applying those skills in a supportive milieu where patients can talk openly about their successes and challenges with the learning process itself. Patients learn from sharing with one another that the learning process is somewhat different for everyone and that there are strategies each individual can use to make the process enjoyable or if not necessarily easier, then at least more palatable. Acting as a facilitator, the group clinician also fosters metacognition by encouraging patients to talk about the skills they use on a given task. Actively 'thinking about one's thinking' tends to stimulate stagnant information-processing systems.

At a more complex level, the group format is also used to stimulate executive functioning, in that some group discussions are devoted to step-by-step problem solving and prioritizing. The group clinician guides patients in a discussion of practical situations (e.g., how to prepare for and get to an appointment with a new doctor) and deconstructs complex tasks so that the whole group engages in helping each other with deliberate problem solving. This type of executive functioning would likely be relatively difficult for patients with chronic cognitive deficits, if they were expected to engage in efficient problem solving spontaneously or otherwise on their own.

Intangible, but nevertheless powerful, benefits of this group work harken back to the tenets of educational psychology, self-determination therapy and client-centered therapy. That is, the bridging group provides patients with a forum for discussion about learning, a way to share learning experiences, to hear the learning experiences of other patients and practice applying cognitive skills. Especially for patients with severe and persistent mental illness and accompanying cognitive deficits, intangible benefits like these can make a difference in humanizing cognitive remediation treatment so that the therapy is more easily tolerated, patients come to treatment more frequently, stay longer and ultimately learn more effectively.

Techniques to Enhance Functional Outcome

As a form of rehabilitation, NEAR is focused on improving cognitive skills in the service of better social role functioning, vocational skills and everyday living skills. To this end, patients are taught not only to have better memory or attention but to then use their better cognitive skills in relevant role situations. To some extent, this requires metacognition ('I need to pay attention when my friend talks'), and to another extent it needs practice. ('Let's help Anna figure out how to get all the jobs done that her bosses requested'). The bridging group provides an excellent forum for both types of role bridging exercise.

In the bridging group, patients learn that improved cognitive skills can make for smoother social transactions and improved social role functioning in a range of circumstances. For instance, there may be discussion of how improved auditory and visual attention to spoken words, facial expressions, tone of voice and gestures can improve one's ability to interact with people in various contexts. On a more complex social-emotional level, such as being a better friend, it helps to attend to words and emotions carefully so that one can more fully acknowledge and support another's experiences and feelings. These are just some examples of the way that bridging groups link cognitive skills specifically to enhanced social role functioning so that improvements in cognitive remediation skills performed on a computer are applied in everyday functioning.

In addition, the group format can provide the very valuable opportunity for patients to practice cognitive skills in various complex cognitive tasks encountered in everyday life. For example, group projects like organizing a pot luck dinner, creating a newsletter or making calendars require the use of cognitive skills within a social context. Patients learn to appreciate how cognitive skills are necessary to complete functional tasks and how to use those cognitive skills to function better in the world and interact more effectively. The group also explores the functional necessity or importance of these cognitive skills, so as to avoid unpleasant social and functional consequences. For example, forgetting names of peers can hurt their feelings and alienate them, and missing doctors' appointments makes it difficult to benefit from medication on a consistent basis, which results in the risk of decompensation or relapse. Patients put their cognitive skills into action in group discussion, by sharing individual experiences with learning, and doing group problem-solving exercises that provide step-by-step ways to deconstruct a psychosocial task (e.g., invite three friends to a weeknight dinner at your home), prioritize and accomplish the component steps.

In both the bridging group and computer-based sessions, opportunities also exist for relatively more experienced patients to assist others in a peer leadership role. Rolling admission to groups means that the group includes patients at all skill levels, from beginner to advanced. Those who have already completed a series of cognitive remediation training may have improved in some cognitive skill areas enough to help other patients with cognitive tasks and take on the role of a peer leader. Peer leaders, while relatively comfortable with some cognitive tasks, may still need improvement developing their own social skills. Helping a peer allows the peer leader to gain self-confidence, self-esteem and practice social skills. The patient who receives assistance from the peer leader has the opportunity to obtain extra instruction and interact with a peer who was helped by the program. The peer leader becomes a heartening, real-life symbol of hope to beginners who may be struggling to figure out how they will productively manage their illness and become the kind of person they want to be.

Finally, group-based cognitive remediation programs create a physical space where patients gather weekly. This regularly scheduled assembly creates its own kind of community among patients who may otherwise be living in relative social isolation due to symptoms of their illness. Besides a sense of community, NEAR's therapeutic milieu provides patients with a sense of safety and support instead of fear or embarrassment. Learning with others who suffer from illnesses of a similar magnitude or severity level also helps patients see how their peers struggle with and address some of the same or related issues involved in the process of rehabilitation and recovery.

Conclusion

The purpose of this chapter was to give an example of how NEAR, which is one of many efficacious approaches to cognitive remediation, targets both cognitive and role functioning. The theories that support NEAR were described to trace its foundations back to seminal theoretical models in neuropsychology, rehabilitation psychology, educational psychology, self-determination theory and client-centered therapy. The chapter describes NEAR's two core treatment components and explains how both individualized cognitive training and bridging group exercises work hand in hand to enhance cognition and social outcomes in daily life at home, at school, at work and in the community.

References

1 Green MF, Kern RS, Braff DL, Mintz J: Neurocognitive deficits and functional outcome in schizophrenia: are we measuring the 'right stuff'? Schizophr Bull 2000;26:119–136.

2 Milberg WP, Hebben N, Kaplan E: The Boston Process Approach to Neuropsychological Assessment; in Grant I, Adams KM (eds): Neuropsychological Assessment of Neuropsychiatric Disorders. New York, Oxford University Press, 1996, pp 65–86.

3 Ben Yishay Y, Diller L: Cognitive rehabilitation in traumatic brain injury: update and issues. Arch Phys Med Rehabil 1993;74:204–213.

4 Sohlberg MM, Mateer CA: Cognitive Rehabilitation. An Integrative Neuropsychological Approach. New York, Guilford Press, 2001.

5 Ben Yishay Y, Prigatano G: Cognitive remediation; in Griffith ER, Rosenthal M, Bond MR, Miller JD (eds): Rehabilitation of the Adult and Child with Traumatic Brain Injury. Philadelphia, Davis, 1990, pp 393–409.

6 Frank RG, Elliott TR: Rehabilitation psychology: hope for a psychology of chronic conditions; in Frank RG, Elliott TR (eds): Handbook of Rehabilitation Psychology. Washington, American Psychological Association, 2000, pp 3–8.

7 Diller L: Neuropsychological rehabilitation; in Meier M, Benton A, Diller L (eds): Neuropsychological Rehabilitation. Edinburgh, Livingstone, 1987, pp 3–17.

8 Kern, RS, Green MF, Mintz J, Liberman RP: Does 'errorless learning' compensate for neurocognitive impairments in the work rehabilitation of persons with schizophrenia? Psychol Med 2003;33:433–442.

9 Bandura A: Self-Efficacy. The Exercise of Control. New York, Freeman, 1997.

10 Schunk DH: Self-efficacy and education and instruction; in Maddux E (ed): Self-Efficacy, Adaptation, and Adjustment. Theory, Research, and Adaptation. New York, Plenum Press, 1995, pp 281–303.

11 Wigfield A, Eccles JS (eds): Development of Achievement Motivation. San Diego, Academic Press, 2002.

12 Cordova DI, Lepper MR: Intrinsic motivation and the process of learning: Beneficial effects of contextualization, personalization, and choice. J Ed Psychol 1996;88:715–730.

13 Kinzie MB: Motivational and achievement effects of learner control over content review within CAI. J Ed Comp Res 1992;8:101–114.

14 Terrell S, Rendulic P: Using computer-managed instructional software to increase motivation and achievement in elementary school children. J Res Comp Ed 1996;26:403–414.

15 Deci EL, Koestner R, Ryan RM: A meta-analytic review of experiments examining the effects of extrinsic rewards on intrinsic motivation. Psychol Bull 1999;125:627–668.

16 Williams GC, McGregor HA, Sharp D, Levesque C, Kouides RW, Ryan RM, Deci EL: Testing a self-determination theory intervention for motivating tobacco cessation: supporting autonomy and competence in a clinical trial. Health Psychol 2006;25: 91–101.

17 Ryan RM, Deci EL: Self-determination theory and the facilitation of intrinsic motivation, social development, and well-being. Am Psychol 2000;55:68–78.

18 Rogers CR: The interpersonal relationship in the facilitation of learning; reprinted in Kirschenbaum H, Henderson VL (eds): The Carl Rogers Reader. London, Constable, 1967/1990.

19 Medalia A, Revheim N, Herlands T: Cognitive Remediation for Psychological Disorders, Therapist Guide. New York, Oxford University Press, 2009.

20 Reeder C, Smedley N, Butt K, Bogner D, Wykes T: Cognitive predictors of social functioning improvements following cognitive remediation for schizophrenia. Schizophr Bull 2006;32:S123–S131.

21 Wykes T, Newton E, Landau S, Rice C, Thompson N, Frangou S: Cognitive remediation therapy (CRT) for young early onset patients with schizophrenia: an exploratory randomized controlled trial. Schizophr Res 2007;94:221–230.

Alice Medalia, PhD
Columbia University College of Physicians and Surgeons
180 Fort Washington Ave., HP 234
New York, NY 10032 (USA)
Tel. +1 212 305 3747, Fax +1 212 305 4724, E-Mail am2938@columbia.edu

Roder V, Medalia A (eds): Neurocognition and Social Cognition in Schizophrenia Patients. Basic Concepts and Treatment. Key Issues Ment Health. Basel, Karger, 2010, vol 177, pp 118–144

5.2

Integrated Psychological Therapy and Integrated Neurocognitive Therapy

Daniel R. Müller · Volker Roder

University Hospital of Psychiatry Bern, Bern, Switzerland

Abstract

This chapter contains 2 examples of combined group therapy approaches for schizophrenia patients: the integrated psychological therapy (IPT) and one of its further developments, the integrated neurocognitive therapy (INT), both initially designed in our laboratory in Switzerland. IPT represents one of the first comprehensive, manual-driven cognitive-behavioral treatment approaches combining cognitive remediation and the improvement of social competence. INT is a newly developed therapy program actually evaluated in an ongoing international randomized controlled trial. It combines neurocognitive and social cognitive enhancement based on the cognitive domains defined by the National Institute of Mental Health- Measurement and Treatment Research to Improve Cognition in Schizophrenia (NIMH-MATRICS) initiative. In this chapter therapists and researchers find information about empirically based theoretical framework, implementation as well as an overview of didactics and exercises of IPT and INT.

The diagnosis of schizophrenia often implies a poor functional outcome [1, 2] responsible for long treatment and high costs of care [1, 3]. Two thirds of the schizophrenia patients suffer from a deterioration of social functioning, even after remission from psychotic symptoms. Social dysfunction is a source of great distress for patients as well as family members [4]. Therefore, the consumer-oriented recovery movement promoted by the mental health commission of the USA included the (re-)establishing of social functioning as one of the main topics in psychiatric rehabilitation of schizophrenia patients [5–8].

Today, new research has provided increasing empirical evidence that the functional outcome is strongly affected by the level of cognitive disturbance in schizophrenia patients [e.g. 9–13]. Cross-sectional analyses of the cognitive impacts using empirical models revealed that the relationship of basic neurocognition (attention, memory, executive functions) and functional outcome is mediated by social cognition [emotion and social perception, theory of mind (ToM), social schema and attribution] [14–18]. Therefore, cognitive impairments are a core feature in schizophrenia, actually discussed to become diagnosis criteria in DSM-V and ICD-11 [e.g. 19]. Cognitive impairments represent a rate-limiting factor in social functioning as well as in the general therapy process and progress with schizophrenia patients. Since psychopharmacological interventions failed to improve cognitive functioning sufficiently in the Clinical Antipsychotic Trial of Intervention Effectiveness study [19], psychological interventions to enhance neurocognition and social cognition became a central therapy target [20]. The psychological intervention best suited to reach this aim is cognitive remediation. On the background of evidence-based medicine, an intervention has to find empirical evidence for its therapy rationale (theory) as well as for its efficacy in laboratory-based, randomized controlled trials and its effectiveness in various standard care settings. Up to date, meta-analyses including randomized controlled trials generally support the efficacy of cognitive remediation in proximal, cognitive outcome [21, 22]. However, only studies that combined cognitive remediation with psychiatric rehabilitation (e.g. therapy of social competence, work rehabilitation) also obtained significant improvements in functional (distal) outcome [22].

Treatment Concept of IPT

On this background, the development of and research on IPT offers some pioneer achievement. IPT was one of the first comprehensive group treatment approaches for schizophrenia patients. The therapy concept of IPT is based on the underlying assumption that basic deficits in cognitive functioning have a pervasive effect on higher levels of behavioral organization (pervasiveness hypothesis [23]). First of all, a link is made between deficits in neurocognitive functioning and the microsocial level, which describes nonverbal and verbal communication in social interactions. This process refers to what is now called social cognition. According to the model of pervasiveness, the link is continued to the macrosocial level of social functioning, i.e. taking over a specific role in the family, job or community. In accordance with vulnerability-stress approaches [24], this model describes that basic neurocognitive deficits lead to difficulties in controlling the intensity and the processing of information (molecular level) and finally reduce the tolerance for interpersonal stress, particularly ambiguous or ambivalent forms. This can in turn lead to inappropriate social functioning. Brenner et al. [25] have described these functionally pervasive developments of deficits as vicious circles, one containing the accumulation of different cognitive deficits, the other comprising the reduction of social skills caused by the first circle. From a historical perspective, this basic work on IPT treatment conception was quite innovative for its time, since the first empirical study on IPT was carried out more than 30 years ago [26] and its first therapy manual in German was published more than 20 years ago [27]. During the last decade, generally accepted integrated models for the explanation of schizophrenia functioning and the theoretical framework of newer integrated therapy approaches have been referred to the initial, empirically driven framework of IPT conception [9, 28]. During the last 3 decades, new research findings and models as well as practical and empirical experience with the program (feedback of patients and therapists; results of studies conducted in different countries) were permanently incorporated into the conception and technology of integrated psychological therapy (IPT). More recently, the IPT concept was supplemented with a modified empirically based integrated model [9] focusing on the relationship of neurocognition, social cognition and symptoms with functional outcome. This model has been expanded by the inclusion of patients' treatment orientation, i.e. insight, intrinsic motivation and treatment compliance relevant to successfully coping with independent life [29, 30].

This theoretical framework of IPT based on empirical findings is consequently operationalized into a comprehensive integrated therapy program consisting of 5 subprograms, each with incremental steps. The IPT procedure starts with neurocognitive remediation, followed by interventions to enhance social cognition. IPT integrated social cognition as one of the key intervention topics in schizophrenia long before its initial definition. The first publication in the Medline database mentioning the term social cognition related to schizophrenia dates from 1993 [31]. In a third stage, IPT transforms the work on cognitive functioning into an interpersonal and social context using verbal communication tools bridging the gap between cognitive and social functioning. Finally, social competence is targeted by exercises to improve social skills and to increase patients' mastery in coping with social problems for a more independent living. In all these steps, IPT considers patients' treatment orientation including therapy motivation.

The Implementation of IPT

IPT has been widely adopted, especially in Europe. Recently, the 6th, revised edition of the German IPT manual was published [29]. The manual has been translated into 12 languages. Actually, Hogrefe Publishers prepare the 2nd, totally revised edition in English [30]. IPT is designed as a cognitive-behavioral group therapy approach. A team of a primary therapist and a co-therapist lead a group of 5–8 patients. The main role of the primary therapist is to structure the group sessions and support and encourage the group members using positive reinforcement and strongly focusing on patients' resources. The function of the co-therapist(s) is formally equal to the patients' role. Additionally, the co-therapist serves as a model for the patients and observes group processes to support and encourage weaker patients. Therapists should focus on behavior and be familiar with processes in groups with schizophrenia patients. In general, therapy sessions should be held twice a week. Groups with elderly patients are often of lower frequency. The sessions stretch from 30 to 90 min. It is difficult to define the duration of each subprogram or the whole therapy program in a general manner. The duration mainly depends on the severity and chronicity of the disorder as well as on the patients' motivation. Accordingly, the number of sessions required to complete a particular subprogram varies relative to the group members' abilities to master the therapy activities. To foster the group members' motivation by bringing more variety into the sessions, in the course of the first 3 subprograms activities from 2 separate subprograms may be conducted during the same session.

The original therapy materials have been modified, extended and differentiated, based on experiences made in different therapy groups. The degree of standardization differs according to the demands of the subprograms. It is usually necessary to modify and complete the materials according to the needs of a specific institution and group. The materials available from the authors [30] are intended to be a pool from which the adequate exercises need to be selected specifically and carefully. The conception of the materials is based on the contents of the therapy, whereby the relevant areas of treatment as well as the different categories of emotion played a decisive role. All therapy exercises should begin with materials considered to be emotionally neutral and easy to carry out ('learning principles'). Only once the group members have achieved some mastery of the exercise with emotionally neutral materials, emotionally loaded task stimuli with increased degree of task difficulty can be introduced.

The Five Subprograms of IPT

IPT consists of 5 subprograms (see fig. 1). The program generally starts with the subprogram 'cognitive differentiation' and ends with 'interpersonal problem solving'. The successful and effective implementation of single subprograms depends on the assessment of differential indication and the respective homogeneity of the patient group to treat. Generally, subprograms take place sequentially. Considering the patients' needs, contents of earlier program stages (e.g. cognitive differentiation) are frequently repeated in later stages (e.g. interpersonal problem solving) as booster sessions within further IPT treatment.

Over the course of the program, each subprogram follows some rules, based on learning principles: (1) start with easy tasks and proceed to more complex and difficult ones later on; (2) start with a high level of structure and reduce it in the course of therapy, and (3) avoid emotional, stress-provoking material and interventions at the beginning of each exercise.

First IPT Subprogram: Cognitive Differentiation

The purpose of this subprogram is to improve the basic neurocognitive processes (e.g. attention, verbal memory, cognitive flexibility, concept formation), which are

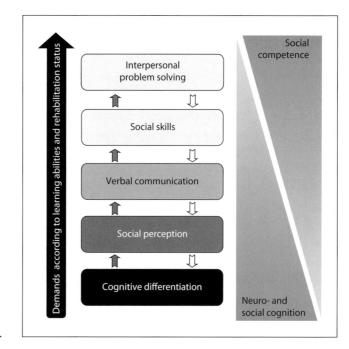

Fig. 1. Schematic presentation of the 5 IPT subprograms.

prerequisites for learning, serving as the cognitive substrates for social interaction and social problem solving. The group format and the consequent support of group interaction throughout all exercises in the subprogram 'cognitive differentiation' distinguishes the IPT procedure from some other neurocognitive remediation approaches: (1) IPT exercises directly address neurocognitive enhancement additionally include a gradually improved training of social cognitions (e.g. emotional processes, ToM, social schema, social attribution) and social skills using group and interpersonal tool; (2) besides the general learning by repeated training of specific neurocognitive skills according to errorless learning principles, IPT focuses strongly on a strategy learning approach to compensate for neurocognitive deficits.

It seems to be optimal to begin with 2-weekly sessions of 30–45 min and to increase the duration to 60 min after a few sessions. The cognitive differentiation subprogram uses a wide variety of exercises. They all comprise 3 steps. Various therapy materials (i.e. cards, worksheets) are available for each step. The group normally progresses from step 1 to step 3 in the sequence described as follows.

Card Sorting Exercises
Each group member obtains a certain number of cards, which are printed with designs that differ in 4 criteria: dimensions of shape, number, days of the week and color (fig. 2). Each participant is asked to sort the cards following the criteria defined by the therapists. Each participant's neighbor then checks to see if the exercise has

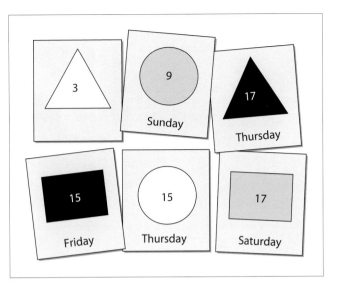

Fig. 2. IPT subprogram cognitive differentiation, step 1: card-sorting exercises.

been done correctly. The level of difficulty is gradually improved by the following repetitions.

Verbal Concept Exercises

There are different exercises for conceptual hierarchies, synonyms, antonyms, word definitions and context-dependent words, which can be carried out with word cards according to the context and exercise.

Conceptual Hierarchy Exercise. Participants are shown a word or phrase (e.g. cooking) and asked to name related words as they come to mind. Afterwards all the words mentioned are organized into hypernyms and hyponyms.

Synonym Exercise. Group members name words with the same meaning as a particular word (e.g. work). They then make up sentences using these words and decide whether there are any differences in meaning.

Antonym Exercise. The procedure is analogous to the synonym exercise.

Word Definition Exercise. The group members are asked to explain a word (e.g. door) to the co-therapist. They try to determine important aspects that enable them to describe the word.

Word Clue Exercise. Group member A is handed a card with 2 words printed on it, of which one is underlined (example: ballpoint pen – <u>fountain pen</u>), and group member A is requested to read both words aloud without revealing which one is underlined. Then he/she is asked to think of a word that enables the other group members to identify the underlined term.

Context-Dependent Word Exercise. The group members explain and discuss the different meanings of a word (e.g. bulb: tulip bulb – light bulb).

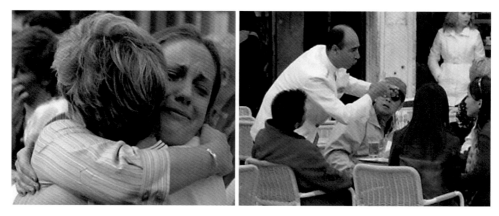

Fig. 3. Examples of slides used in the IPT subprogram social perception.

Object Guessing Exercises

One group member chooses an object in the room. The name of the object is written down for future checking, but this information is not shared with the other group members. The group's task is to determine which object they were thinking of through a series of questions, which can be answered by 'yes' or 'no'. The group members practice asking questions, gradually proceeding from very concrete to conceptual ones. Their use of conceptual questions is encouraged.

Second IPT Subprogram: Social Perception

The social perception subprogram of IPT takes into consideration the contextual and social components of cognitive functioning. The use of therapy materials operationalizes the 2 social cognitive domains, i.e. social perception and affect recognition. The objective of this subprogram is to improve the participant's visual perception of social situations and the emotion involved. Along with cognitive differentiation, the social perception subprogram supports the cognitive enhancement, which represents a precondition for successful acquisition of interpersonal, social and community skills.

The social perception subprogram uses a series of slides depicting social situations. Some of the slides additionally involve facial expression of affect or gestures. The slides, which have been rated for their level of difficulty, vary in visual complexity (number of presented stimuli) and emotional loading. For the 6th German and the 2nd English edition of the IPT manual [30], a completely new set of 40 slides was evaluated (fig. 3). At the beginning of therapy, slides rated with a low degree of complexity and emotional loading are presented. The level of difficulty gradually increases as the group members make progress. The subprogram aims to improve the apprehension and interpretation of social situations and perceived emotions. For this purpose, an important objective is that patients learn to separate between facts and assumptions.

The therapist uses 3 therapeutic steps to work with each slide.

Gathering Information

The group members are asked to describe a slide as accurately and as detailed as possible. At this step the slide should not be interpreted. Gathering information step by step and learning how to describe situations is a fundamental and important objective in this subprogram, building the base of the further proceeding.

Interpretation and Discussion

Group members are asked to state their views on possible interpretations of the situation and the expressed emotions depicted on the slide. Every opinion needs justification by reference to the actual visual information gathered in the first step. All the group members subsequently discuss the different possible interpretations. They learn how to judge the correctness and the likeliness of each interpretation. By comparing and substantiating various interpretations, the participants learn to resolve cognitive dissonance rather than just adopting group consensus. In addition, they learn to decode facial affects and emotional gestures and to understand how and why a social situation can be interpreted in various ways.

Assigning a Title

After gathering information and interpreting the pictures, the therapist asks the group members to choose a title for the picture. It should be short and meaningful, reflecting the most important aspects of the social situation on the slide (summarizing the contents of the slide). The appropriateness of the suggested title will enable the therapists to verify whether the key aspects of a situation have been perceived and understood.

Third IPT Subprogram: Verbal Communication

On the background of the incremental steps within the IPT procedure, the subprogram verbal communication is designed to serve as a bridge between the 2 first subprograms focusing on cognition and the 2 last ones addressing social functioning. The verbal communication subprogram requires patients to use and transfer the learned cognitive skills into interpersonal communication. It focuses on 3 basic communication skills.

Listening

Respecting and attending to other people's contributions to a conversation.

Understanding

Correctly perceiving and interpreting the content of the transmitted information.

Responding
Formulating and sending an appropriate response.

The group members practice these basic skills in 5 consecutive steps. The tasks assigned gradually become more difficult; the demands increase during therapy. Work sheets are available for each step. For the initial phases, the therapy material is highly structured and task oriented, becoming less structured as the therapy progresses. The purpose of this incremental procedure is to help participants acquire more differentiated communication skills, which can eventually be applied to real-life interaction.

Failure to successfully cope with problems at higher levels of therapy indicates that the therapist should go back to the previous level(s). Once the fifth step is reached, the therapist needs to pay additional attention to the way each participant verbally interacts outside the confines of the therapy program. The therapy procedure will subsequently be described step by step.

Literal Repetition Exercise
A group member gets a card with a sentence printed on it and is asked to read it to the group aloud. Another member of the group literally repeats this sentence. All group members check if the exercise is being done correctly.

Paraphrasing Exercise
This exercise resembles step 1, the difference being that on each card only 1 or 2 words are presented. One group member is handed a card and asked to make up his or her own sentence with the words. The other group members then have to reproduce this sentence in their own words, yet retaining its meaning.

W-Question Exercise
The group or the therapist introduces a topic of discussion (e.g. ward, hobby) and writes it down on the blackboard. The group compiles a list of words related to that topic. These words are written down on cards, analogous to step 2. Each group member is asked to choose one of the word cards as well as a question word starting with 'W' (where, when, who, why, etc.), to combine them in a question and to ask it to another group member. The group then monitors if the question is related to the discussion topic and whether the answer refers to the question asked.

Asking Questions about a Topic
The group asks 1 or 2 members questions about a certain topic (e.g. newspaper article). The group members again monitor the process of communication.

Focused Communication Exercise
Once more, the group is provided with a topic of discussion. It can be adopted from newspaper articles, short stories, proverbs or figures of speech, slides or topics of interest

for the group members. The most important aspect of this activity is the evaluation of communication skills. Group members (acting as observers) or the therapists can serve as evaluators. The evaluation should take place on 2 levels. In order to evaluate the quality of the *contents*, the following questions should be asked: 'How well were the contributions understood?' 'How well did the participants respond to what had been said?' 'How high was the quality of what was expressed?' 'Did the participants wander off to unrelated or irrelevant matters?' However, an evaluation of the *nonverbal* aspects of communication should be conducted as well (e.g. eye contact, fluency, loudness, tone of voice, etc.).

Fourth IPT Subprogram: Social Skills

The subprogram social skills follows the enhancement of cognitive functioning as well as the re-establishment of basic conversational skills during the IPT procedure. The acquisition and improvement of social skills represents a precondition for reaching an adequate level of social competence reflecting self-efficacy and real-world success in patients' daily lives. Today it is discussed that deficits in social competence refer to an impaired premorbid social adjustment, which interacts with factors that are adverse to individualization and socialization processes, largely inhibiting social learning. Furthermore, social competence refers to social incompetence, which tends to increase the longer the illness and hospital confinement last. Therapeutic techniques have to help the patient acquire or reactivate an adequate repertoire of social skills. Therefore, working on concrete behavioral aspects on the level of molecular skills such as posture, eye contact, facial expression, gestures, volume of speech and verbal fluency is as important as improving molar, i.e. more complex as well as more highly integrated and sequentially patterned modes of behavior during therapy.

On this background, the social skills subprogram uses certain techniques of behavior therapy such as instruction, modeling, shaping, coaching, role play, feedback and reinforcement. The focus of therapy is put on various social problems participants are confronted with in their daily lives. These include problem areas such as everyday life on the ward or at home, looking for work and accommodation, dealing with authorities, home care, as well as job and leisure skills. The therapy materials include examples of concrete situations addressed to these areas. The social skills training has 2 main purposes. On the one hand, it aims at helping participants generalize therapy gains to a number of real-life situations, and on the other hand, it sets out to meet the patients' needs and to address their particular deficits and impairments. The latter aspect mainly involves cognitive processes and setting up the role play. The therapy procedure implemented in this subprogram comprises 2 steps.

Setting Up the Role Play
The therapist begins the session by explaining the (new) role play to be practiced and the interactional goals. The practice situation should be presented as simply,

clearly and concretely as possible. The group members are encouraged to identify the demands they are confronted with in a particular situation and to elaborate a dialogue. Then they have to assign an appropriate title to the role play. Asking the group to reach a consensus on an appropriate title enables the therapists to verify if the group members have understood and retained the basic points and the interaction goals to be achieved. The next step involves a discussion of anticipated difficulties, which serves to decrease fears and related anxieties. Finally, the group members are asked to rate the perceived level of difficulty of the role play using a scale from 1 (very easy) to 5 (very difficult).

Enacting the Role Play

First of all a small stage area with realistic props is prepared. Then the therapists enact the role play to provide a model for the group members. The participants benefit more if their models are not perfect. A feedback phase follows. First, the 'active therapist' comments on the role play. Then, the group members act as observers making a comment on specific aspects of the role play. The primary therapist should make sure that all their feedback is positive. In the next step, the group members start participating actively in the plays. The participant who originally found the exercise to be particularly easy (i.e. had rated it low in difficulty) begins. The cotherapist keeps his or her role. Feedback is given each time a group member enacts a role. The therapists have various techniques to assist group members (e.g. prompting, coaching). Positive reinforcement is, however, one of the most effective methods. Once the group has become adept at role plays, they may benefit from examining a videotape of their performance. To assist group members in generalizing the social skills they are learning, each therapy session ends with the assignment of a homework exercise (in vivo transfer).

Fifth IPT Subprogram: Interpersonal Problem Solving

Interpersonal problem solving is the final step of the IPT therapy program. It follows the preceding neurocognitive and social cognitive remediation and the increase in social skills. This subprogram sets high demands on the participants: schizophrenia patients sometimes have difficulties in appropriately identifying problems. Especially interpersonal problems in daily life are strongly associated with emotional distress leading to difficulties for the patients in coping adequately. It is important for the participants to acquire factual and problem-oriented attitudes and reasonable ways to solve problems to reduce the risk of failing in everyday life. They should also learn to anticipate the consequences of a solution objectively and unemotionally.

Problem-solving strategies must be applied to real-life situations whenever possible (in vivo transfer). Again, worksheets that address problems in everyday life such as budget, looking for work and accommodation, or home care are available.

The interpersonal problem solving subprogram is comprised of 7 steps following a problem solving model, which need to be conducted in sequence.

Problem Identification and Analysis

In the initial step of interpersonal problem solving, the therapist chooses a problem area to be addressed with the group after having carefully assessed and defined it by interviewing the group members. The problem area to start working with is usually chosen according to its urgency as well as to its probability of finding a solution. It is low in complexity and emotional loading. The principle of gradually increasing the level of emotional distress is acted upon analogously to the other IPT subprograms.

Problem Description

The cognitive description of a problem involves several goals, such as correcting idiosyncratic attitudes, learning to distinguish fact from fiction and how to break down complex problems into integral, well-defined parts of the overall difficulty, identifying the behavioral aspects of a problem and fostering pragmatic attitudes in order to enable a modification of the behavior.

Generating Alternative Solutions

Once the group has successfully described the problem, they can proceed with working out possible alternative solutions. In this phase of the treatment, the therapist encourages the group to come up with as many solutions as possible (brainstorming technique). The therapist reinforces all the suggestions made and notes them. At this point, it is important for the therapist not to assess or judge the suggestions.

Evaluating the Alternatives

Once various alternatives have been found, their advantages and disadvantages are weighed by assigning plus or minus points to each suggestion. The total number of points for each alternative can be calculated. This rating scale enables the group to develop an objective and neutral method of assessment. The therapist should accept emotionally biased judgments or assessments but not reinforce them.

Deciding on a Solution

The group selects an appropriate solution together, according to the previous procedure. However, each patient needs to say which solution best fulfills his/her own needs. The therapist's job is to decide to what extent he/she should influence the decision-making process.

Translating the Solution into Action

Once a solution has been selected, the most difficult step of therapy follows, namely the translation of the chosen solution into action. Numerous *therapeutic measures* ranging from in vivo exercises to residential training programs can help the participants attain the goals of this subprogram. However, a solution can only be considered valid if it proves of value in real-life situations. Whenever possible a role play for a solution should be performed.

Feedback Sessions

The participants report the experiences they have made with the designated solution. Each attempt at constructive problem solving should be encouraged. Failing to solve a problem should not be interpreted as a reason for resignation. It should much rather motivate the patient to correct the designated problem-solving behavior. Such feedback sessions can substantially contribute to a lasting therapy success. Working on a 'problem' can require a period of several therapy sessions. Meticulously preparing the sessions and keeping strict record of them can, however, save a considerable amount of time.

Evaluation of IPT

Besides the broad implementation of the IPT technology in Europe, America and Asia, a large body of evaluation studies was conducted by independent research groups in 12 countries. Research was carried out with in- and outpatients in randomized controlled trial and field studies taking place in academic and nonacademic sites. Thirty-four investigations were quantitatively reviewed in a meta-analysis including 1,515 patients [3]. To our knowledge, IPT represents the first and only therapy approach for schizophrenia patients which was exclusively the object of a meta-analysis. The results suggest significant effects of IPT in various proximal and distal outcomes independently of the setting, site condition and quality of the trial. These favorable IPT effects compared to controls are the result of the specific interventions rather than of group treatments alone: in the control conditions, unspecific group activities to control the group effect showed stronger influences compared with treatment as usual in social cognition, social functioning and negative symptoms but not in neurocognition. However, IPT groups showed superior effects compared to both control conditions. Furthermore, the detailed analysis of IPT subprograms indicated an additional benefit for the combined interventions using the neuro- and social cognitive IPT subprograms in cognitive and functional outcome compared to the use of the neurocognitive subprogram alone [32]. A variety of studies on IPT used only single subprograms or a combination of subprograms. In accordance with the theoretical framework of IPT, only studies based on the complete IPT program generated sufficient generalization effects and were maintained from the end of treatment to follow-up [3, 32]. In summary, there is strong evidence for the efficacy and effectiveness of IPT. The American Psychological Association Task Force on Serious Mental Illness and Severe Emotional Disturbance classifies IPT as a state-of-the-art intervention and includes it in the Catalog of Clinical Training Opportunities: Best Practice for Recovery and Improved Outcomes for People with Serious Mental Illness (available at: http://www.apa.org/practice/smi_grid-v2.pdf; accessed June, 2009).

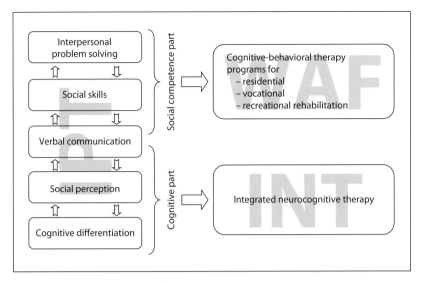

Fig. 4. Further development of IPT subprograms.

Further Developments of IPT

In order to capitalize on advances made in intervention technology and therapy topics associated with an improved understanding of schizophrenia functioning, the IPT concept was expanded and modified in our laboratory in Bern. In 2 research projects supported by the Swiss National Foundation our research group developed and evaluated 2 new therapy approaches: the 3 cognitive social skill programs for residential, vocational and recreational topics (WAF; grant No.: 32–45577.95) and the integrated neurocognitive therapy (INT; grant No. 3200 3B–108133) for schizophrenia patients (see fig. 4).

First of all, the scope of the IPT subprograms social skills and interpersonal problem solving was extended by developing 3 cognitive social skill programs for residential, vocational and recreational topics (we use the German abbreviation for 'Wohnen, Arbeit, Freizeit', WAF, [33]). The 3 WAF programs introduce rehabilitation topics that are particularly relevant to schizophrenia patients. Therefore, WAF represents cognitive and behavioral interventions to improve social competence in specific functional areas of patients' daily lives instead of a general, rather unspecific support of social functioning used in IPT. Patients are treated with only 1 WAF therapy program depending on indication. The groups usually comprise 6–8 participants guided by a therapist and a cotherapist. Each of the 3 WAF programs focuses on (a) sensitizing the patients to their needs, options and skills (cognitive and emotional skill training); (b) helping them make a decision in any of these 3 areas; (c) providing support in putting the decision taken into action (practical implementation of skills), and (d) teaching them how to anticipate difficulties and to solve concrete problems. All 3 programs have the same structure, which on the whole allows for flexible behavior and problem analysis. WAF was evaluated in an international multicenter study including 143 schizophrenia patients. The results suggested additional effects of WAF compared to traditional social skill therapy in proximal outcome (find a competitive job, leisure time activities, change in less structured housing offers) and a symptom reduction. Additionally, a relapse reduction was evident in a 5-year follow-up [33–36].

Integrated Neurocognitive Therapy

In a second step, our research group revised the basic IPT subprograms cognitive differentiation and social perception and designed the INT. An empirically based starting point for the development of INT came from IPT and WAF evaluation: a combination of the neurocognitive and social cognitive IPT subprogram yielded superior effects in proximal and distal outcome compared to neurocognitive remediation alone [32, 37]. Intrinsic motivation represented a strong mediator of improved functional outcome in the WAF procedure [35–37], which is in line with data derived from other research studies [38–40]. Following the IPT technology, the primary aim of the development of INT was to integrate neurocognitive and social cognitive exercises using group processes as therapeutic tools. Therefore, INT as well as IPT decisively differ from laboratory-based traditional cognitive remediation approaches. Another aim is the orientation to patients' individual resources rather than their deficits.

Treatment Concept of INT

Based upon the theoretical and empirical state of neurocognitive and social cognitive research described earlier in this book, we developed a cognitive-behavioral group therapy approach. For this purpose, the original IPT model was modified. Conceptually, INT is built upon the definitions of the National Institute of Mental Health MATRICS initiative (Measurement and Treatment Research to Improve Cognition in Schizophrenia) [41–43]. Following the recommendations of this task force, 6 neurocognitive domains (speed of processing, attention/vigilance, verbal and visual learning and memory, working memory, as well as reasoning and problem solving) and 5 social cognitive domains (emotional processing, social perception, ToM, social schema and attribution style) were operationalized for therapeutic intervention.

The Implementation of INT

INT is designed as cognitive-behavioral group therapy in outpatient settings. A team of a primary therapist and a cotherapist lead a group of 6–8 patients. The roles and

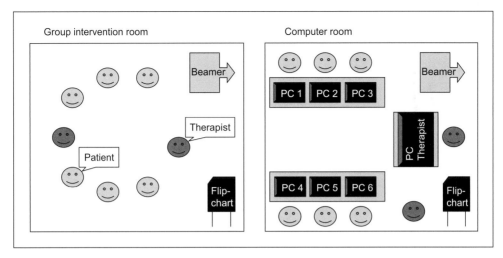

Fig. 5. Infrastructure needed for the INT.

functions of the therapy team are the same as described in the IPT section. A total of 30 sessions are administered. They take place biweekly and each last 90 min including a short break. Due to the outpatient setting, the exercises and therapy content are designed to have higher demands on patients' capacity and competence in a group setting compared to IPT. A not yet published manual for the use in a multicenter research project is available [37]. It includes a broad scope of interventions in neurocognitive and social cognitive domains offering the therapists to compose exercises according the participants' needs.

Since INT also includes computer-based exercises, the therapy procedure requires a computer room in addition to the standard group intervention room (fig. 5). During a therapy session of 90 min, the PC-based exercises are limited to 45 min. Therefore, patients and therapists have to switch from the specially equipped PC room to the group intervention room during each session. In the group as well as in the PC-based exercises group processes are used as basic therapeutic tools. In an ongoing international randomized-controlled evaluation study, the Cogpack computer program distributed by Marker Software is used.

The Four Subparts (Modules) of INT

INT consists of 4 therapy subparts (modules), each including different functional domains of neurocognition and social cognition. A schematic presentation of INT is given in figure 6.

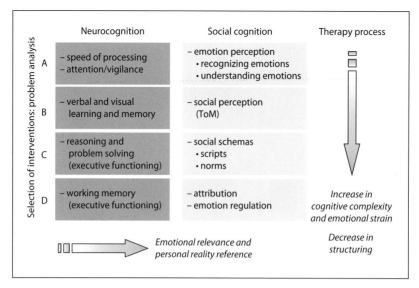

Fig. 6. Schematic presentation of the INT.

Based on an integrated model [9, 30] confirmed by recent empirical data [14–17, 44–47], social cognition mediates the relationship between neurocognitive capacities and the acquisition of social skills as well as a generalization to the broad level of social functioning. Consequently, the inclusion of social cognitive therapy tools and the reference to patients' experience of their cognitive functioning during daily living increase the emotional relevance and additionally support the generalization of proximal treatment effects to the level of social functioning. Furthermore teaching patients cognitive functions and their relevance in real-life situations within a vulnerability-stress-coping framework of schizophrenia enhances their insight into individual cognitive capacity. Individualized coping strategies (compensatory approach) are derived to compensate difficulties in daily life. Therefore, INT places a strong emphasis on fostering patients' intrinsic therapy motivation. The reinforcement of the cognitive resources in repeated practice exercises using errorless learning principles as well as new experiences of successful coping in daily life enhances self-efficacy expectancy in terms of creating a sense of self-empowerment. Following the IPT tradition, the sequence of the INT subparts follows explanatory models describing mechanisms of interaction between basic and more complex cognitive skills with higher emotional strain [25, 48]. In accordance with the IPT program, the level of structuring group processes decreases during therapy.

This 'bottom up' and 'top down' approach puts a strong focus on the patients' daily life context to promote transfer and generalization. Enhancing insight into (illness-specific) cognitive resources and deficits, as well as possibilities of coping represents

Table 1. Therapy components of each of the 4 INT modules (subparts)

Each treatment area (A–D) of INT comprises:
- Introduction sessions
  Perception of personal resources and possibilities of optimizing them in daily life
  Education in the focused therapy area (→ 'insight' into problems/deficits)
  → Use of case vignettes
- Consecutive sessions
  Compensation: looking for coping strategies
  Restitution: practicing exercises (rehearsal)
  → Partly computer-based

For all therapy components: in vivo exercises and homework assignments to promote transfer and generalization.

a further aim of treatment. All 4 modules include the same didactic therapy components (table 1).

In each module, INT starts with introduction sessions using educational tools to support patients' understanding of the focused cognitive domain and its relevance in daily life. A precondition to bridge the gap between the experiences made in the laboratory during therapy and the daily living context outside the laboratory is to establish the patients' awareness of their own resources and to enhance their insight into deficits in cognitive functions and their corresponding limitations in coping with daily problems. For this purpose, prototypical case vignettes (short stories) were designed for each cognitive domain. In these stories, the same imaginary actors always have successful or unsuccessful experiences based on specific cognitive resources or deficits. As a first step, the introduction of a theme through the use of these short stories gives patients as a first step the opportunity to discuss cognitive functioning without a relation to their own often stressful, emotionally loaded experiences. In a second step, the patients are asked whether they have had experience in daily life similar to the content of the stories.

In the consecutive sessions in each INT module, individual coping strategies are elaborated in the group setting. They compensate for cognitive deficits and optimize the individual resources for managing the demands of daily life associated with cognitive functioning. In parallel with this strategy learning approach, the INT procedure includes repeated training sessions, which are partially PC based. In this rehearsal approach, a large body of exercises is group based, using group processes and interactions to activate patients and to simulate real-life situations. Also during a computer session, therapists largely support group processes. For example, they ask patients to argue and discuss their solution as well as to articulate possible strategies in team competition. Finally, in vivo exercises and homework assignments are used to promote transfer of the learned cognitive skills into practice, to support generalization of the effects to other functions and to maintain the effects after therapy.

Module A of INT

After a short overview of the contents of the INT procedure, information-processing models are used to elucidate the impact of cognitive functioning on daily living. In this context, patients are asked about their own perceived resources and deficits in general cognitive functioning for the first time. Then, INT starts with the introduction of the basic neurocognitive domains of speed of processing and attention, followed by the social cognitive domain of emotion perception. In the beginning, the INT procedure is very structured and the cotherapist is working as a model in each new exercise.

Speed of Processing
Very simple PC-based exercises are introduced to give patients confidence in handling the computer. The level of difficulty is augmented following errorless learning principles. Additionally, behavioral therapy techniques such as positive reinforcement and positive connotation are implemented to support patients' motivation and self-efficacy expectancy. Afterwards, patients' experiences during the PC exercises are discussed in the group context. A strong focus is given to the identification of patients' individual resources and deficits in this functional area. The relevance of speed of processing in daily living situations is summarized for each participant. Furthermore, patients learn coping strategies to compensate for deficits and to optimize resources by the didactic use of information and work sheets. Information sheets summarize the knowledge about the function of speed of processing in information processes and behavior. The work sheets individualize the information by asking patients whether they have any experience in dealing with such problems at work, in leisure time activities or at home. Finally, the learned compensation strategies are habituated in repeating the PC exercises of the introduction session.

Attention
Alertness and vigilance are addressed separately. Both are introduced by reading prototypical short stories in the group. Again, PC-based exercises addressing attention functioning in understimulating tasks are repeatedly practiced. In a following educational part, patients learn that speed and attention functioning is strongly affected by the state of mood and the level of interest. Here, newly developed card-sorting exercises are introduced to combine possibilities of emotional expression and the level of attention using verbal stimuli.

Emotion Perception
This topic was already introduced in the neurocognitive part of module A using the card-sorting exercise described above referring to the intention of INT to always intervene in neurocognition and social cognition in parallel. A filter model addressing the relationship

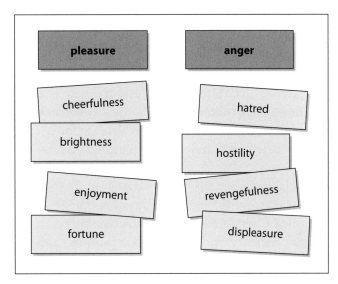

Fig. 7. INT module A: example of card-sorting exercise addressing emotional concept formation.

of perception and memory and individual experience introduces perceptual processes. Therein, emotional distress and mood are declared as a possible filter. Patients are asked about their own or others' experience with each of these basic emotions. For a better understanding of the emotional impact, the relationship of emotional feeling to neurocognitive functioning, somatic reaction and behavior is explored in patients' daily living experience.

A large body of pictures from the IPT, from other sources or from new sets standardized in our laboratory is available in the manual to train affect decoding. Here, the INT procedure starts with unambiguous pictures including simple stimuli of facial affect, followed by pictures addressing facial affect and gestures, and ends with complex pictures showing emotionally loaded interpersonal situations.

In complementing affect recognition tasks, a second card sorting exercise was designed to address emotional concept formation: patients receive dark and light grey cards. One basic emotion is written on each of the dark grey cards. The light grey cards contain different commonly used terms, most concerning 1 basic emotion. Others are ambiguously referring to more than 1 emotion. The patients have to sort the cards according to the basic emotions (fig. 7). Each decision has to be argued to find a group consensus. If this is not possible due to the ambiguous meaning of a word, 2 solutions are accepted. Finally, the impact of the emotional state on cognitive functioning in daily life in terms of the use of speech is discussed in the group.

Module B of INT

Didactically, the second module of INT is strongly related to the content of module A. The already introduced filter model explains the relationship between perception and memory, wherein the quality of selective attention of the environment is postulated as strongly dependent on individuals' earlier experience and mood. The 2 MATRICS dimensions verbal learning and memory, and visual learning and memory are dealt with separately, beginning with the former. The social cognitive part of this module represents a straight continuation of the perceptual process introduced in module A. The patients learn to recognize the key information in social situations. On this background, INT works on patients' assumption of other's intention and thinking in a social situation, which is defined in the literature as Theory of Mind (ToM).

Verbal Learning and Memory
This neurocognitive domain is introduced by reading 2 prototypical short stories in the group. One short story addresses the short-term memory, the other one the prospective memory. Again, the relevance of the personal level of functioning in this area to cope with life successfully and patients' assumptions are focused. Patients first train memory skills in repeated PC-based exercises using errorless learning strategies. Thereafter, patients' experience of their performance in the PC exercises is compared with their estimation made before to identify their resources and deficits in verbal memory. Following a normalizing approach, deficits and resources are positively connotated: everybody has an individual profile of cognitive functioning comprising parts of strength and weakness; it is hardly possible to have strength in every domain of cognitive functioning. Individual strategies of the patients used in daily living to compensate for these deficits are summarized and completed through handouts. Information sheets are available for the short-term as well as for the prospective memories. The compensation strategies are exercised in the repetition of the PC tasks. Additionally, we developed group exercises to simulate real-life situations and to force group processes. For example, in a role play in which all patients participate, every patient gets a card including the name, the hobby and the favorite color of a fictive person, e.g. a politician, or a popular movie or sports star. In a highly structured exercise, each patient reads the warrant of the respective person on his/her card, which has to be memorized by the other group members. Such exercises, which probably take participants' interests of private life into account, strongly support the motivation for active participation in the program.

Visual Learning and Memory
The intervention on visual learning follows the same steps as described for verbal learning and memory. Working on visual learning is less time-consuming than working on verbal learning; too much repetition should be avoided. The contents of PC-based exercises include traffic signs and other figurative cues instead of verbal tasks.

Social Perception
The intervention in this cognitive domain is strongly based on the one used in the IPT procedure. For example the same series of pictures of the IPT is used. Additionally, a

set of more complex pictures was designed to augment the level of difficulty. Some of the contents of the pictures are taken into action using role plays. This helps to activate the patients and gives them an experience of the key aspects of the situation.

Theory of Mind

As mentioned above, ToM functioning is stimulated in a group setting per se. In the social perception task before, ToM skills were already trained implicitly by the interpretation of depicted interpersonal situations. On this background, we developed the following exercise: the group is split into 2 parts. While 1 half leaves the room together with the cotherapist doing some alternative exercises, the other half chooses a picture out of a set of landscapes and describes the chosen one in detail analogous to the social perception task (sending group). The members of the sending group memorize the detailed description. The other half of the group returns to the room without knowing the targeted picture. Then the sending group verbalizes the description and the members of the other group (receiving group) have to take over the verbalized perspective to form an internal picture. This should help the receiving group recognize the targeted picture from the set. In further exercises, the participants have to take over the perspective of actors in fictive written stories, movies or comics. Some of the contents of these ToM exercises are also transferred into role plays. Thereby, the emotional impact of the actors and the comparison with individual daily life experience are of special interest.

Module C of INT

Module C focuses on the MATRICS domains of reasoning and problem solving representing the highest level on neurocognitive demands. The 2 targeted domains are dealt with separately, beginning with reasoning. The social cognitive part of this module addresses social schemas including exercises on social norms and social scripts.

Reasoning

The module starts with reading a short story concerning the targeted cognitive function in a social context. In the educational part, the term 'reasoning' is replaced by 'thinking' in the context of daily living situations. A strong focus is given to patients' own thoughts in dependence on concrete social situations and its emotional impact. Moreover, the verbal communication skills in interpersonal behavior represent an intervention topic by the use of verbal concept tasks: PC-based exercises are followed by group exercises concerning conceptual hierarchies like in the IPT procedure. On an advanced level patients improve their capacity to find the right words during a communication and to summarize in their own words what they have experienced when watching a movie or reading a book. Additionally, the competence in planning a certain behavior is taken into consideration. Again, this is operationalized in a group exercise: the course of concrete actions well known in daily living, such as cooking spaghetti or going to a birthday party, is split apart into sequences. The therapist writes these sequences on different cards. Each patient gets 1 card. The group members have to put the different cards (sequences) in the right order.

Problem Solving

A standard problem-solving model commonly used in cognitive-behavioral therapy is taught. The patients then repeat abstract laboratory-based computer exercises for problem solving. These exercises are partly done in small groups of 2 or 3 patients to emphasize group interaction and the social context of problem solving. The patients have to argue and convince the other group members of their own solution and have to find a consensus. Riddles are used as well. In another group session, each patient mentions a problem he/she actually could not solve. The problems should be rather simple with a high possibility of finding a solution during therapy (e.g. to clean the apartment, to find a friend). The standard problem-solving techniques are applied (compare IPT).

Social Schemas

Many techniques described in 'reasoning and problem solving' are used, but social relations stay in the foreground. Social schemas are modified in 2 ways: first by the use of social action sequences (scripts) and second by the reflection of the impact given trough social norms and roles. For instance, in a social script exercise 4 cards with pictures referring to a common daily action (e.g. buying a bus ticket; ordering a meal) are presented to the group. The patients then describe the pictures on the cards and afterwards they try to get the cards (sequences) into the right order. Finally the patients find a title best describing the content of the sequence. Again, they are instructed to use facts and not assumptions to argue.

Module D of INT

Finally, the last module addresses working memory. While the topic of the first module was understimulation derived by sensory poverty, this part completes the INT concept with topics referring to overstimulation associated with sensory overload. The working memory comprises therapy sessions concerning cognitive flexibility and selective attention processing. Emotional strain associated with stressfully experienced overstimulation and possibilities of coping are a main focus during the sessions. Additionally, social cognitive interventions include the impact of the individual attribution style to emotionally loaded stress features – often associated with psychotic positive symptoms. Consequently, patients' emotional strain is highest in this final part of the INT procedure. On this background, it seems necessary that emotional as well as behavioral coping strategies are implemented.

Working Memory

In the first educational part, the patients read a short story wherein the protagonist has to shift between several actions during a competitive work. The cognitive flexibility skills needed are related to personal experiences of the participants. Compensation strategies are introduced using information sheets. The following intervention uses work sheets to individualize and transfer the coping compensation strategies into concrete daily living situations. With the help of PC-based exercises the patients first train the learned strategies on a high abstraction level. Role plays then stimulate the use of cognitive flexibility skills in a social context before each patient tries to implement the learned skills in his personal area. In a second short story, the patients learn that coping with a stress-inducing sensory overloaded situation demands selective attention skills. All exercises analyze cognitive, emotional, behavioral and somatic consequences of internal and external overstimulation. Introducing a vulnerability-stress-coping model, patients learn to understand how individual stress is preconditioned and how to manage stressful situations. Thereby, the impact of the environment, interpersonal and social circumstances, as well as individual resources are considered. In a final stress inoculation training the patients learn to cope with stress.

Attribution

Many schizophrenia (out-)patients suffer from persistent positive symptoms associated with negative life experiences. The social cognitive domain of attribution is often strongly related to positive symptoms. In appraising a situation, schizophrenia patients often jump to conclusions without gathering all the information or show an overgeneralized attribution. Thus, intervening in attribution can lead to a high emotional strain for the patients. This is the reason why INT addresses this theme at the end, when the group has established high cohesion (friendship and confidence). Here, INT works with standardized descriptions of concrete situations. The fictive protagonist, who is well known from the short stories read in the group, acts in situations taken out of real life. The probability is high that some patients have had comparable experiences. For example, 'Peter (fictive protagonist) is sitting in a restaurant drinking a coffee and reading a newspaper. A man eating at another table looks at him from time to time.' The patients are asked to describe the situation and to formulate hypotheses why the man is looking at Peter. All alternative hypotheses are summarized and evaluated. The cognitive, emotional and behavioral consequences of each hypothesis are analyzed. The patients are drilled to consequently use facts instead of assumptions and that facts have to be completed before the situation can be interpreted. The described situation is then practiced in role plays to stimulate patients' perception of related feelings. This represents 1 goal of the INT procedure: that patients experience their feelings related to a concrete situation and that a change in thinking and behavior has emotional consequences.

Feasibility of INT

In an ongoing randomized multicenter study, supported by the Swiss National Foundation, 8 centers in Switzerland, Germany and Austria participate. Up to now, a total of 145 schizophrenia outpatients could be included. In this project, the feedback given by therapists and patients was excellent. The low dropout rate of only 11% and the relatively high rate of over 80% of optional session participation indicate a high acceptance of the INT procedure by patients. The first study results show a superior proximal outcome in the cognitive area compared to treatment as usual. Additionally, these favorable effects could be generalized to a more distal outcome of social functioning and negative symptoms. These therapy effects could be maintained during a follow-up of 1 year [49]. Consequently, INT represents a new promising cognitive remediation approach which seems to be feasible and effective.

References

1 Wittorf A, Wiedemann G, Buchkremer G, Klingberg S: Prediction of community outcome in schizophrenia 1 year after discharge from inpatient treatment. Eur Arch Psychiatry Clin Neurosci 2008;258:48–58.

2 Addington J, Addington D: Social and cognitive functioning in psychoses. Schizophr Res 2008;99:176–181.

3 Roder V, Müller DR, Mueser KT, Brenner HD: Integrated Psychological Therapy (IPT) for schizophrenia: is it effective? Schizophr Bull 2006;32(suppl 1):81–93.

4 Bellack AS, Green MF, Cook JA, Fenton W, Harvey PW, Heaton RK, Laughren T, Leon AC, Mayo DJ, Patrick DL, Patterson TL, Rose A, Stover E, Wykes T: Assessment of community functioning in people with schizophrenia and other severe mental illnesses: a white paper based on an NIMH-sponsored workshop. Schizophr Bull 2007;33:805–822.

5 Liberman RP, Kopelowicz A: Recovery from schizophrenia: a concept in search and research. Psychiatr Serv 2005;56:735–742.

6 Bellack AS: Scientific consumer models of recovery in schizophrenia: concordance, contrasts, and implications. Schizophr Bull 2006;32:432–442.

7 Leucht S, Lasser R: The concepts of remission and recovery in schizophrenia. Pharmacopsychiatry 2006;39:161–170.

8 Lieberman JA, Drake RE, Sederer LI, Begler A, Keefe R, Perkins D, Stroup S: Science and recovery in schizophrenia. Psychiatr Serv 2008;59:487–496.

9 Green MF, Nuechterlein KH: Should schizophrenia be treated as a neurocognitive disorder? Schizophr Bull 1999;25:309–318.

10 Milev P, Ho BC, Arndt S, Andreasen NC: Predictive values of neurocognition and negative symptoms on functional outcome in schizophrenia: a longitudinal first-episode study with 7-year follow-up. Am J Psychiatry 2005;162:495–506.

11 Cohen AS, Leung WW, Saperstein AM, Blanchard JJ: Neuropsychological functioning and social anhedonia: results from a community high-risk study. Schizophr Res 2006;85:132–141.

12 Matza LS, Buchanan R, Purdon S, Brewster-Jordan J, Zhao Y, Revicki DA: Measuring changes in functional status among patients with schizophrenia: the link with cognitive impairments. Schizophr Bull 2006;32:666–678.

13 Bowie CR, Reichenberg A, Patterson TL, Heaton BK, Havey PD: Determinants of real-world functional performance in schizophrania subjects: correlations with cognition, functional capacity, and symptoms. Am J Psychiatry 2006;163:418–425.

14 Vauth R, Rusch N, Wirtz M, Corrigan PW: Does social cognition influence the relation between neurocognitive deficits and vocational functioning in schizophrenia. Psychiatry Res 2004;128:155–165.

15 Brekke J, Kay DD, Lee KS, Green MF: Biosocial pathways to functional outcome in schizophrenia. Schizophr Res 2005;80:213–225.

16 Sergi MJ, Rassovsky Y, Nuechterlein KH, Green MF: Social perception as a mediator of the influence of early visual processing on functional status in schizophrenia. Am J Psychiatry 2006;163:448–454.

17 Bell M, Tsang HWH, Greig TC, Bryson GJ: Neurocognition, social cognition, perceived social discomfort, and vocational outcomes in schizophrenia. Schizophr Bull 2009;35:738–747.

18 Keefe RSE: Should cognitive impairment be included in the diagnostic criteria for schizophrenia? World Psychiatry 2008;7:22–28.

19 Keefe RSE, Bilder RM, Davis SM, Harvey PD, Palmer BW, Gold JM, Meltzer HY, Green MF, Capuano G, Stroup TS, McEvoy JP, Swartz MS, Rosenheck RA, Perkins DO, Davis CE, Hsiao JK, Lieberman JA: Neurocognitive effects of antipsychotic medications in patients with chronic schizophrenia in the CATIE trial. Arch Gen Psychiatry 2007;64:633–647.

20 Green MF: Cognition, drug treatment, and functional outcome in schizophrenia: a tale of two transitions. Am J Psychiatry 2007;164:992–994.

21 Pfammatter M, Junghan UM, Brenner HD: Efficacy of psychological therapy in schizophrenia: conclusions from meta-analyses. Schizophr Bull 2006; 32(suppl 1):64–80.

22 McGurk SR, Twamley EW, Sitzer DI, McHugo GJ, Mueser KT: A meta-analysis of cognitive remediation in schizophrenia. Am J Psychiatry 2007;164: 1791–1802.

23 Brenner HD: Zur Bedeutung von Basisstörungen für Behandlung und Rehabilitation; in Böker W, Brenner HD (eds): Bewältigung der Schizophrenie. Bern, Huber, 1986.

24 Zubin J, Spring BJ: Vulnerability – A new view of schizophrenia. J Abnorm Psychol 1977;86:103–126.

25 Brenner HD, Hodel B, Roder V, Corrigan P: Treatment of cognitive dysfunctions and behavioral deficits in schizophrenia: Integrated Psychological Therapy. Schizophr Bull 1992;18:21–26.

26 Brenner HD, Stramke WG, Mewes J, Liese F, Seeger G: Erfahrungen mit einem spezifischen Therapieprogramm zum Training kognitiver und kommunikativer Fähigkeiten in der Rehabilitation chronisch schizophrener Patienten. Nervenarzt 1980;51:106–112.

27 Roder V, Brenner HD, Kienzle N, Hodel B: Integriertes Psychologische Therapieprogramm (IPT) für schizophrene Patienten. München, Psychologie Verlags-Union, 1988.

28 Hogarty GE, Flesher S, Ulrich R, Carter M, Greenwald D, Pogue-Geile M, Kechavan M, Cooley S, DiBarry AL, Garrett A, Parepally H, Zoretich R: Cognitive enhancement therapy for schizophrenia: effects of a two-year randomized trial on cognition and behavior. Arch Gen Psychiatry 2004;61:866–876.

29 Roder V, Brenner HD, Kienzle N: Integriertes Psychologisches Therapieprogramm bei schizophren Erkrankten IPT. Weinheim, Beltz, 2008.

30 Roder V, Mueller DR, Spaulding W, Brenner HD: Integrated Psychological Therapy for Schizophrenia Patients (IPT). Goettingen, Hogrefe, 2010.

31 Corrigan PW, Green MF: Schizophrenic patients' sensitivity to social cues: the role of abstraction. Am J Psychiatry 1993;150:589–594.

32 Mueller DR, Roder V: Empirical evidence for group therapy addressing social perception in schizophrenia; in: Teiford JB (ed) Social Perception. 21st Century Issues and Challenges. New York, Nova Science Publishers, 2008, pp 51–80.

33 Roder V, Zorn P, Pfammatter M, Andres K, Brenner HD, Mueller DR: Praxishandbuch zur verhaltenstherapeutischen Behandlung schizophren Erkrankter, ed 2, rev. Bern, Huber, 2008.

34 Roder V, Brenner HD, Mueller D, Laechler M, Zorn P, Reisch T, Bösch J, Bridler R, Christen C, Jaspen E, Schmidl F, Schwemmer V: Development of specific social skills training programmes for schizophrenia patients: results of a multicentre study. Acta Psychiatr Scand 2002;105:363–371.

35 Roder V, Mueller DR, Zorn P: Therapieverfahren zu sozialen Fertigkeiten bei schizophren Erkrankten in der Arbeitsrehabilitation. Vorteile des Aufbaus arbeitsspezifischer gegenüber unspezifischer sozialer Fertigkeiten. Z Klin Psychol Psychother 2006; 35:256–266.

36 Mueller DR, Roder V: Social skills training in recreational rehabilitation of schizophrenia patients. Am J Recreational Ther 2005;4:11–19.

37 Roder V, Mueller DR: Integrated Neurocognitive Therapy (INT) for Schizophrenia Patients (unpublished manual). Bern, University Psychiatric Hospital, 2006.

38 Medalia A, Lim RW: Self-awareness of cognitive functioning in schizophrenia. Schizophr Res 2004; 71:331–338.

39 Medalia A, Richardson R: What predicts a good response to cognitive remediation interventions? Schizophr Bull 2005;31:942–953.

40 Nakagami E, Xie B, Hoe M, Brekke JS: Intrinsic motivation, neurocognition and psychosocial functioning in schizophrenia: testing mediator and moderator effects. Schizophr Res 2008;105:95–104.

41 Green MF, Nuechterlein KH: The MATRICS initiative: developing a consensus cognitive battery for clinical trials. Schizophr Res 2004;72:1–3.

42 Nuechterlein KH, Barch DM, Gold JM, Goldberg TE, Green MF, Heaton TE: Identification of separable cognitive factors in schizophrenia. Schizophr Res 2004;72:29–39.

43 Green MF, Olivier B, Crawley JN, Penn DL, Silverstein S: Social cognition in schizophrenia: recommendations from the Measurement and Treatment Research to Improve Cognition in Schizophrenia New Approaches Conference. Schizophr Res 2005; 31:882–887.

44 Brüne M: Emotion recognition, 'Theory of Mind', and social behavior in schizophrenia. Psychiatry Res 2005;133:135–147.

45 Addington J, Saeedi H, Addington D: Facial affect recognition: a mediator between cognitive and social functioning in psychosis? Schizophr Res 2006;85: 142–150.

46 Pinkham AE, Penn DL: Neurocognitive and social cognitive predictors of interpersonal skill in schizophrenia. Psychiatry Res 2006;143:167–178.

47 Sergi MJ, Rassovsky Y, Widmark C, Reist C, Erhart S, Braff DL, Marder SR, Green MF: Social cognition in schizophrenia: relationships with neurocognition and negative symptoms. Schizophr Res 2007;90:316–324.

48 McGurk SR, Mueser KT: Cognitive functioning, symptoms and work in supported employment: a review and heuristic model. Schizophr Res 2004;72: 147–173.

49 Roder V, Mueller DR: Remediation of neuro- and social cognition: results of an international randomized multi-site study. Schizophr Bull 2009; 35(suppl 1):353–354.

Prof. Volker Roder
University Hospital of Psychiatry
Bolligenstrasse 111
CH–3000 Bern 60 (Switzerland)
Tel. +41 31 930 99 07, Fax +41 31 930 99 88, E-Mail roder@sunrise.ch

Roder V, Medalia A (eds): Neurocognition and Social Cognition in Schizophrenia Patients. Basic Concepts and Treatment. Key Issues Ment Health. Basel, Karger, 2010, vol 177, pp 145–157

6

Pharmacological Interventions

Alex Hofer · W. Wolfgang Fleischhacker

Department of Psychiatry and Psychotherapy, Biological Psychiatry Division, Medical University Innsbruck, Innsbruck, Austria

Abstract
Cognitive deficits have highly consistent relationships to overall morbidity in schizophrenia patients and exert a greater influence on community functioning and the ability to acquire skills in psychosocial rehabilitation than the presence or severity of positive or negative symptoms. Accordingly, there is considerable interest in finding psychopharmacological therapies in addition to psychosocial interventions for treating the cognitive deficits intrinsic to the disorder. The currently available antipsychotic medications do not have sufficient cognitive effects for meaningful improvements. There has therefore been a continued need for improved treatment of these impairments. Here we review potential molecular targets that are actively explored, including dopamine, serotonin, adrenergic, muscarinic and nicotinic acetylcholine receptors, the glutamatergic excitatory synapse, and the γ-aminobutyric acid system.

The clinical picture of schizophrenia was described for the first time by the German physician Emil Kraepelin who used the term 'dementia praecox' to define a disorder with an early beginning, a uniformly deteriorating course and a poor prognosis [1]. Although this term already characterized the relationship between cognitive deficits and schizophrenia more than a century ago, effective treatments for these disorders have not yet been developed.

Today, the cognitive impairments in schizophrenia are considered to be core features of the illness, and they have been shown to lack correlation with the severity of positive symptoms and to be only mildly correlated with the severity of negative symptoms. Furthermore, they relate directly to sociovocational functioning and exert a greater influence on both the ability to acquire skills in psychosocial rehabilitation and functional outcome than the presence or severity of positive or negative symptoms. In addition, the severity of cognitive deficits is considered predictive of medication compliance and overall treatment adherence.

Ninety percent of the patients with schizophrenia are estimated to have clinically meaningful deficits in at least 1 cognitive domain, and 75% have deficits in at least 2

[2]. Such cognitive disturbances are present both in children who have a schizophrenic parent ('high-risk children') and in first-degree relatives of patients who do not suffer from a schizophrenic disorder. Cognitive deficits are clearly present in the first episode of the illness, even in antipsychotic-naïve patients, and thus are not a deleterious effect of treatment. Furthermore, they are apparent long before the onset of psychotic symptoms and they endure after a psychotic episode when patients are in remission. Therefore, cognitive deficits represent a possible trait marker of schizophrenia.

Generally, it is assumed that schizophrenia patients show deficits across a large number of neurocognitive domains including working memory, speed of processing, verbal learning and memory, attention and vigilance, reasoning and problem solving, and visual learning and memory [3]. On average, performance has been reported to be 1.5 to 2.5 standard deviations below population norms on standardized psychometric tests, consistent with mild to moderate cognitive impairment, and even those patients who perform within age-adjusted norms [2] exhibit cognitive abilities below those expected if they did not have the disease.

Next to neurocognitive impairment schizophrenia has consistently been associated with deficits in social cognition (i.e. emotion perception, social perception, theory of mind, attributional style) [3]. Studies have shown a consistent relationship between social cognition and various domains of functional outcome. In addition, next to measures of functional capacity (i.e. key tasks of daily living such as preparation of meals or management of medications) measures of social cognition have been shown to act as mediators between neurocognition and functional outcome in schizophrenia [4].

The Neuropharmacology of Cognition in Schizophrenia

Due to the strong association between cognitive impairment and functional disability, there is considerable activity and interest from both academia and the pharmaceutical industry in developing therapies to enhance cognition in schizophrenia. Clearly, the discovery of first generation antipsychotics in the early 1950s represented a medical and scientific landmark as it was for the first time possible to treat the positive symptoms of schizophrenia. These treatments, however, are generally not thought to be very effective at treating the negative and cognitive symptoms of schizophrenia which may be one possible reason for the lack of improvement in outcome associated with these older compounds. There is some evidence that first generation antipsychotic drugs improve some aspects of attentional functioning, while mild negative effects have been noted on some measures of motor speed and on procedural learning, which appears to be attributable to extrapyramidal side effects and adjunctive anticholinergic agents, which are known to impair memory and global cognitive performance. Furthermore, patients treated with first generation antipsychotic medications do not show the level of practice-related improvements shown by healthy individuals when tested repeatedly [5]. There is some evidence for the superiority of new generation antipsychotics over first generation compounds in improving cognitive performance [6, 7], but the effect size of these differences was not large (in the range of 0.2–0.4 standard deviations) and the results were inconsistent. Furthermore, studies had methodological limitations: the sample size of some of these trials was small and they did not always account for relevant confounders such as other symptom improvement, anticholinergic treatment, change in extrapyramidal symptoms, and practice. Of interest, more recent studies using lower doses of the first generation compounds found smaller differences between first and new generation medications than earlier studies [8, 9]. It has therefore been suggested that the use of a relatively high dose of the first generation drug as the comparator might have biased earlier results in favor of the new generation antipsychotic drugs. These methodological issues have been adressed by the Clinical Antipsychotic Trials of Intervention Effectiveness study [10] that has investigated chronically ill patients and by the European First-Episode Schizophrenia Trial [11]. The Clinical Antipsychotic Trials of Intervention Effectiveness study reported that although cognitive performance improved in all groups during treatment with olanzapine, perphenazine, quetiapine, risperidone and ziprasidone, there were no statistically significant differences among the groups after 2 and 6 months of treatment. At 18 months, the cognitive improvement was greatest in the perphenazine group [12]. Similarly, the European First-Episode Schizophrenia Trial reported on moderate neurocognitive improvements in patients with schizophreniform disorder or those who were in the first episode of schizophrenia after 6 months of treatment with either low-dose haloperidol, amisulpride, olanzapine, quetiapine or ziprasidone. Again, there were no differences among the 5 treatment groups [13]. Hence, it has been suggested that the size of the difference in neurocognitive effects between first- and new-generation compounds may depend partly on the dose of the first-generation antipsychotic. Similar considerations may also apply to the effects of antipsychotic medications on social cognition. For example, Kee et al. [14] reported a benefit for risperidone compared to 15 mg of haloperidol in this regard, while Sergi et al. [15] did not find any significant changes in social cognition in patients treated with either olanzapine, risperidone or 8 mg of haloperidol. Direct head-to-head comparisons of new-generation antipsychotics did not find any significant difference between treatments with regard to their cognitive effects either [16].

Taken together, the development of antipsychotic medications has had a profound effect on the treatment of schizophrenia, but the cognitive deficits associated with this disorder have been insufficiently addressed. It is therefore critical to continue the search for novel pharmacological approaches to achieve meaningful gains in this regard. The following molecular targets for drug development have been identified: dopamine, serotonin, adrenergic, muscarinic and nicotinic acetylcholine receptors, the glutamatergic excitatory synapse, and the γ-aminobutyric acid (GABA) system.

Dopaminergic Approaches

Dopamine D_1 Receptors

It has been hypothesized that decreased dopaminergic neurotransmission in the prefrontal cortex may contribute to the cognitive impairments observed in schizophrenia, especially those related to working memory and executive functioning. Indeed, the majority of the prefrontal dopamine receptors are of the D_1 subtype, and a decrease in dopamine-D_1-receptor-like binding in the prefrontal cortex has been found to correlate with the severity of cognitive dysfunction in schizophrenia patients. On the other hand, subcortical mesolimbic dopamine D_2 pathways have been shown to be disinhibited and overactive in schizophrenia, and dopamine antagonists are known to be therapeutic for positive symptoms. However, in nonhuman primates, chronic blockade of D_2 receptors by antipsychotic drugs leads to a downregulation of D_1 receptors in the prefrontal cortex and consequently runs the risk of exacerbating cognitive impairments. There is thus a strong rationale for evaluating the potential efficacy of dopamine D_1 agonists in patients with schizophrenia. Indeed, selective D_1 agonists enhance cognitive functioning in nonhuman primates and reverse the cognitive deficits in monkeys treated chronically with a D_2 receptor antagonist [17, 18]. However, chronic treatment with D_1 agonists may actually lead to the downregulation of D_1 receptors potentially worsening cognition in the long term. Furthermore, clinical research with direct-acting D_1 agonists has been hindered by their propensity to induce hypotension secondary to peripheral D_1 stimulation, which may necessitate the use of indirect D_1-activating agents such as catechol-O-methyltransferase (COMT) inhibitors (see below). Nevertheless, dihydrexidine, a full D_1 agonist, is now undergoing preliminary investigation in patients with schizophrenia and has not produced significant blood pressure drop so far [19] while enhancing perfusion in D_1-populated cortical regions relevant to cognition [20].

Dopamine D_4 Receptors

Despite the high affinity of clozapine for dopamine D_4 receptors that had led to the speculation of particular pathophysiolical relevance of D_4 receptors, clinical trials of selective D_4 antagonists did not demonstrate any appreciable efficacy in the treatment of acute schizophrenia. However, D_4 blockade could improve cognition by decreasing N-methyl-D-aspartate (NMDA) receptor activity in the hippocampus [21] and by inhibiting glutamatergic signaling in the prefrontal cortex [22], while D_4 agonists may suppress $GABA_A$ inhibitory currents in the prefrontal cortex and thereby indirectly enhance cortical excitability [23]. Therefore, D_4-receptor-selective compounds may be valuable in the treatment of the cognitive deficits in schizophrenia.

Catechol-O-Methyltransferase

COMT regulates prefrontal information processing by means of deactivation of dopamine through methylation and is therefore known to have an effect on prefrontally mediated cognitive functioning. Interestingly, genetic variation in COMT has been shown to be a key mechanism involved in prefrontal dopamine metabolism. Concretely, the Val allele, because of its higher capacity to metabolize dopamine, has been associated with a relatively compromised frontal function, while the Met allele has been found to result in greater availability of prefrontal dopamine and, thus, to be linked to some aspects of cognition [24]. Accordingly, several studies have identified an association between working memory and executive functioning, and COMT the Va1108/158Met genotype in schizophrenia. Furthermore, Met homozygous and Val/Met heterozygous patients demonstrate significantly greater cognitive response to clozapine than Val homozygous patients [25].

These studies underline the role of dopamine and COMT in the modulation of prefrontal cortex activity and suggest potential benefits of COMT inhibitors for the treatment of cognitive disorders associated with impaired prefrontal functioning, especially in individuals with Val/Val alleles because of their higher enzyme activity. Indeed, tolcapone, a selective reversible inhibitor of COMT, has been reported to improve cognitive dysfunction in patients with advanced Parkinson's disease [26] and provides a valuable tool for the treatment of cognitive disorders in patients with schizophrenia.

Serotonergic Approaches

5-HT$_{2A}$ Receptors

Apart from involvement in attention, learning and memory, serotonin (5-hydroxytryptamine, 5-HT) is known to play a key role in mood and emotion as well as a number of psychiatric conditions including depression, anxiety and schizophrenia. For example, an interaction with 5-HT$_{2A}$ receptors has been associated with the cognition-enhancing effects of new-generation antipsychotics, probably through normalization of NMDA receptor functionig [27] and modulation of dopaminergic tone, particularly along the mesocortical pathway [28]. Accordingly, administration of mianserin, a 5-HT$_{2A/2C}$ and α_2-adrenergic antagonist, has been shown to improve cognitive functioning in schizophrenia patients [29]. However, it is unlikely that coadministration of 5-HT$_{2A}$ antagonists to treatment with new-generation antipsychotics with inherent 5-HT$_{2A}$ antagonistic actions will provide any significant boosting of cognition [30].

5-HT$_{1A}$ Receptors

Among others, the 5-HT$_{1A}$ receptor antagonism of some new-generation antipsychotics (e.g. risperidone, sertindole) has been associated with cognition-enhancing effects, probably due to facilitation of glutamatergic transmission [31]. On the other hand, the 5-HT$_{1A}$ receptor partial agonism of other new-generation antipsychotics (e.g. aripiprazole, clozapine, olanzapine, quetiapine, ziprasidone) has been suggested to enhance the release of dopamine and acetylcholine in the prefrontal cortex and hippocampus [32] and to alter the release of glutamate and GABA [33], thereby improving cognitive functioning as well. Similarly, chronic administration of tandospirone, a 5-HT$_{1A}$ partial agonist, has been shown to enhance executive functioning and verbal learning and memory in patients with schizophrenia treated with first-generation antipsychotics, while buspirone augmentation of treatment with new generation antipsychotics led to improvements in attention/speeded motor performance [34].

5-HT$_6$ Receptors

The affinity of the HT$_6$ receptor for certain antipsychotics (e.g. clozapine, olanzapine) as well as antidepressant drugs (e.g. amitriptyline, clomipramine) supports the hypothesis that 5-HT$_6$ ligands may have a therapeutic role in neuropsychiatric conditions. Various neurochemical studies indicate that 5-HT$_6$ receptor antagonists modulate excitatory amino acid, dopamine and acetylcholine neurotransmission and may therefore have memory-enhancing capabilities [35]. Indeed, the 5-HT$_6$ receptor antagonist SB-271046 has been shown to improve acquisition and recall in the water maze test in rats [36]. Consequently, HT$_6$ receptors may have an important future role in the treatment of cognitive deficits in neuropsychiatric illnesses.

5-HT$_7$ Receptors

As in the case of the HT$_6$ subtype, HT$_7$ receptors also bind several antipsychotics (e.g. clozapine, risperidone) and antidepressant drugs (e.g. mianserine, maprotiline) with high affinity [35]. Based on receptor distribution (hippocampus, thalamus, hypothalamus) and preliminary pharmacologic analyses, it has been suggested that the HT$_7$ receptor might represent another serotonergic target for memory enhancement [37] and might therefore prove therapeutically useful for the treatment of cognitive dysfunction in schizophrenia.

Hofer · Fleischhacker

α₂-Adrenergic Receptors

α₂-Receptor agonists have been shown to be effective in preventing many of the behavioral, neurochemical and anatomical effects of NMDA antagonists, probably due to an attenuation of enhanced dopamine release, and to inhibit excitatory synaptic transmission in the prefrontal cortex, thereby enhancing working memory [38]. In schizophrenia patients, treatment with clonidine and guanfacine has demonstrated some improvements in cognitive performance without exacerbating positive symptoms, especially in those treated with new-generation antipsychotics [39, 40]. However, by preferentially enhancing dopaminergic transmission in the frontal cortex over subcortical dopaminergic pathways, α₂-receptor *antagonism* has been associated with the atypicality of some new-generation antipsychotics (e.g. clozapine) [41]. It is therefore challenging to balance α₂-receptor activity to achieve both antipsychotic and procognitive efficacy.

Cholinergic Approaches

Next to its role in motor functioning the cholinergic system has been implicated in the regulation of various domains of cognition, particularly attention, learning and memory [42]. Accordingly, decreased nicotinic and muscarinic acetylcholine receptors in the cortex and hippocampus of schizophrenia patients [43, 44] might contribute to their cognitive deficits.

Acetylcholinesterase Inhibitors

In recent years, there have been several trials of acetylcholinesterase inhibitors in patients with schizophrenia, but they have not been overly supportive of this approach. Overall, galantamine appears to be more clinically promising for an enhancement of verbal memory and processing speed than other acetylcholinesterase inhibitors such as donezepil and rivastigmine, probably due to its additional action as a positive allosteric modulator of the $\alpha_4\beta_2$- and α_7-nicotinic receptors [45–47]. Therefore, the modulation of various subtypes of both nicotinic and muscarinic acetylcholine receptors may be a more effective approach to treat the cognitive impairment in schizophrenia. However, a 12-week, double-blind, placebo-controlled trial of galantamine as adjunctive treatment to first-generation antipsychotic drugs found no significant improvement in the Mini-Mental State Examination or psychiatric symptoms [48]. Similarly, in another placebo-controlled add-on study [49] a high dose of galantamine was well tolerated but not effective against cognitive deficits.

Nicotinic Receptors

It is well known that the smoking rates in patients with schizophrenia are significantly higher than in the general population, an observation that has sometimes been explained as an attempt at self-medication. Generally, nicotine improves some aspects of cognition in schizophrenia patients, especially in nonsmokers [50]. However, treatment with agonists at α_7-nicotinic receptors is not effective due to rapid desensitization of nicotinic receptors [51, 52]. Therefore, partial agonists and allosteric potentiators (e.g. galantamine) of α_7-nicotinic receptors might represent potential alternatives due to minimal induction of receptor desensitization.

Muscarinic Receptors

Next to the ionotropic nicotinic receptors, various studies have implicated metabotropic muscarinic acetylcholine receptors in schizophrenia, especially the M_1 subtype [53]. For example, postmortem studies have found decreased M_1 receptor binding in the prefrontal cortex, hippocampus and striatum of patients with schizophrenia [54]. This alteration has been suggested to contribute to the cognitive dysfunction intrinsic to this disorder. Accordingly, M_1 receptor agonism might be beneficial in treating these deficits. It has been assumed that the cognitive enhancement observed with clozapine could actually be due to its metabolite N-desmethylclozapine, a potent M_1 agonist. Similarly, treatment with xamomeline, among other actions a nonselective M_1 and M_4 muscarinic agonist, led to an improvement in positive symptoms and cognitive functioning, though this compound was discontinued due to poor tolerability [55].

Glutamatergic Approaches

Glutamate mediates its CNS effects via both ionotropic and metabotropic receptors. Ionotropic receptors are differentiated upon sensitivity to the synthetic glutamate derivatives NMDA, α-amino-3-hydroxy-5-methyl-4-isoxazolepropionic acid (AMPA) and kainate. The NMDA receptor antagonists phencyclidine and ketamine are known to produce a wide range of schizophrenia-like symptoms, including positive, negative and cognitive ones. It has therefore been hypothesized that some deficiency in NMDA functioning might play a role in the pathophysiology of schizophrenia and that augmentation of NMDA receptor activity might consequently have therapeutic potential. It has also been proposed, however, that some symptoms of schizophrenia result from rebound hyperglutamatergia secondary to primary NMDA blockade, leading to seemingly contradictory pharmacologic approaches being explored [56].

NMDA Receptors: Glycine Site Agents

Direct agonists of the glutamate-binding site of the NMDA receptor may not be clinically feasible due to the risk of excess excitation causing neurotoxicity and seizures. Therefore, the allosteric glycine-binding site has been targeted for drug development in schizophrenia. In general, full agonists, such as glycine and D-serine, have proven more effective than D-cycloserine, likely due to it being a partial agonist that acts as an antagonist at high doses. However, in a recently conducted study neither glycine nor D-cycloserine could be demonstrated to improve negative symptoms or cognition [57]. Furthermore, these drugs have not shown clinical efficacy when added to clozapine, suggesting that clozapine's unique therapeutic effects may be due its ability to enhance glycine and glutamate neurotransmission [58].

NMDA Receptors: Glycine Transport Inhibitors

Another approach to treatment is the use of glycine transport inhibitors to increase synaptic glycine levels by preventing neuronal and glial uptake. Use of the low-potency glycine transport inhibitor sarcosine led to a highly significant reduction in negative symptoms, along with smaller but significant reductions in positive and cognitive symptoms in both patients with chronic schizophrenia stabilized on first- or new- generation antipsychotics [59] and acutely decompensated subjects [60]. Similarly to studies with direct glycine site agonists, no beneficial effects of sarcosine were observed in patients treated with clozapine [61].

AMPA Receptors

AMPA receptors work synergistically with NMDA receptors and are needed to maintain the overall integrity of glutamate synapses. Direct AMPA receptor agonists lead to a rapid desensitization of AMPA receptors limiting their therapeutic utility. Therefore, allosteric AMPA receptor modulators, termed ampakines, which have been found to facilitate learning and memory in animal models and in preliminary trials in human subjects, were studied as potential treatments for schizophrenia. However, they were not found to be effective for cognition or for other symptoms of schizophrenia when added to new-generation antipsychotics [62].

GABAergic Approaches

Among others, prefrontal cortical impairments in schizophrenia are thought to reflect a deficiency in the synchronization of pyramidal cell activity that is dependent, in part, on GABA neurotransmission through receptors containing α_2-subunits. Accordingly, agents that stimulate the α_2-subunit have been proposed as a pharmacological strategy for treating cognitive dysfunction. Indeed, MK-0777, a benzodiazepine-like agent with selective activity at GABA$_A$ receptors containing α_2- or α_3-subunits, has recently been shown to improve working memory function in schizophrenia patients [63]. Further clinical trials are needed to explore this novel treatment strategy for schizophrenia.

Conclusion

Cognitive impairment is a core feature of schizophrenia and is a determinant of the daily functioning of patients. The utility of available antipsychotics, however, is limited in this regard. Thus, optimal treatment of schizophrenia currently relies on individualized polypharmacy and augmentation strategies, highlighting the strong need for continued basic research efforts at identifying and validating novel molecular targets in order to advance outcomes beyond remission of psychosis and toward functional recovery.

References

1 Kraepelin E: Psychiatrie. Ein Lehrbuch für Studierende und Ärzte, ed 4. Leipzig, Abel, 1893.

2 Palmer BW, Heaton RK, Paulsen JS, Kuck J, Braff D, Harris MJ, Zisook S, Jeste DV: Is it possible to be schizophrenic yet neuropsychologically normal? Neuropsychology 1997;11:437–446.

3 Nuechterlein KH, Barch DM, Gold JM, Goldberg TE, Green MF, Heaton RK: Identification of separable cognitive factors in schizophrenia. Schizophr Res 2004;72:29–39.

4 Brekke JS, Kay DD, Kee KS, Green MF: Biosocial pathways to functional outcome in schizophrenia. Schizophr Res 2005;80:213–225.

5 Mishara AL, Goldberg TE: A meta-analysis and critical review of the effects of conventional neuroleptic treatment on cognition in schizophrenia: opening a closed book. Biol Psychiatry 2004;55:1013–1022.

6 Harvey PD, Keefe RS: Studies of cognitive change in patients with schizophrenia following novel antipsychotic treatment. Am J Psychiatry 2001;158:176–184.

7 Woodward ND, Purdon SE, Meltzer HY, Zald DH: A meta-analysis of neuropsychological change to clozapine, olanzapine, quetiapine, and risperidone in schizophrenia. Int J Neuropsychopharmacol 2005;8:457–472.

8 Green MF, Marder SR, Glynn SM, McGurk SR, Wirshing WC, Wirshing DA, Liberman RP, Mintz J: The neurocognitive effects of low-dose haloperidol: a two-year comparison with risperidone. Biol Psychiatry 2002;51:972–978.

9 Keefe RS, Seidman LJ, Christensen BK, Hamer RM, Sharma T, Sitskoorn MM, Lewine RR, Yurgelun-Todd DA, Gur RC, Tohen M, Tollefson GD, Sanger TM, Lieberman JA: Comparative effect of atypical and conventional antipsychotic drugs on neurocognition in first-episode psychosis: a randomized, double-blind trial of olanzapine versus low doses of haloperidol. Am J Psychiatry 2004;161:985–995.

10 Lieberman JA, Stroup TS, McEvoy JP, Swartz MS, Rosenheck RA, Perkins DO, Keefe RS, Avis SM, Davis CE, Lebowitz BD, Severe J, Hsiao JK; Clinical Antipsychotic Trials of Intervention Effectiveness (CATIE) Investigators: Effectiveness of antipsychotic drugs in patients with chronic schizophrenia. N Engl J Med 2005;353:1209–1223.

11 Fleischhacker WW, Keet IP, Kahn RS; EUFEST Steering Committee: The European First Episode Schizophrenia Trial (EUFEST): rationale and design of the trial. Schizophr Res 2005;78:147–156.

12 Keefe RS, Bilder RM, Davis SM, Harvey PD, Palmer BW, Gold JM, Meltzer HY, Green MF, Capuano G, Stroup TS, McEvoy JP, Swartz MS, Rosenheck RA, Perkins DO, Davis CE, Hsiao JK, Lieberman JA; CATIE Investigators; Neurocognitive Working Group: Neurocognitive effects of antipsychotic medications in patients with chronic schizophrenia in the CATIE Trial. Arch Gen Psychiatry 2007;64: 633–647.

13 Davidson M, Galderisi S, Weiser M, Werbeloff N, Fleischhacker WW, Keefe RS, Boter H, Keet IP, Prelipceanu D, Rybakowski JK, Libiger J, Hummer M, Dollfus S, López-Ibor JJ, Hranov LG, Gaebel W, Peuskens J, Lindefors N, Riechler-Rössler A, Kahn RS: Cognitive Effects of Antipsychotic Drugs in First-Episode Schizophrenia and Schizophreniform Disorder: A Randomized, Open-Label Clinical Trial (EUFEST). Am J Psychiatry 2009;70:717–729.

14 Kee KS, Kern RS, Marshall BD, Green MF: Risperidone versus haloperidol for perception of emotion in treatment-resistant schizophrenia: preliminary findings. Schizophr Res 1998;31:159–165.

15 Sergi MJ, Green MF, Widmark C, Reist C, Erhart S, Braff DL, Kee KS, Marder SR, Mintz J: Social cognition and neurocognition: effects of risperidone, olanzapine, and haloperidol. Am J Psychiatry 2007; 164:1585–1592.

16 Keefe RS, Sweeney JA, Gu H, Hamer RM, Perkins DO, McEvoy JP, Lieberman JA: Effects of olanzapine, quetiapine, and risperidone on neurocognitive function in early psychosis: a randomized, double-blind 52-week comparison. Am J Psychiatry 2007; 164:1061–1071.

17 Cai JX, Arnsten AF: Dose-dependent effects of the dopamine D_1 receptor agonists A77636 and SKF81297 on spatial working memory in aged monkeys. Psychopharmacology 1997;283:183–189.

18 Castner SA, Williams GC, Goldman-Rakic PS: Reversal of antipsychotic-induced working memory deficits by short-term dopamine D_1 receptor stimulation. Science 2000;287:2020–2022.

19 George MS, Molnar CE, Grenesko EL, Anderson B, Mu Q, Johnson K, Nahas Z, Knable M, Fernandes P, Juncos J, Huang X, Nichols DE, Mailman RB: A single 20-mg dose of dihydrexidine (DAR-0100), a full dopamine D_1 agonist, is safe and tolerated in patients with schizophrenia. Schizophr Res 2007;93: 42–50.

20 Mu Q, Johnson K, Morgan PS, Grenesko EL, Molnar CE, Anderson B, Nahas Z, Kozel FA, Kose S, Knable M, Fernandes P, Nichols DE, Mailman RB, George MS: A single 20-mg dose of the full D_1 dopamine agonist dihydrexidine (DAR-0100) increases prefrontal perfusion in schizophrenia. Schizophr Res 2007;94:332–341.

21 Kotecha SA, Oak JN, Jackson MF, Perez Y, Orser BA, Van Tol HH, MacDonald JF: A D_2 class dopamine receptor transactivates a receptor tyrosine kinase to inhibit NMDA receptor transmission. Neuron 2002;35:1111–1122.

22 Rubinstein M, Cepeda C, Hurst RS, Flores-Hernandez J, Ariano MA, Falzone TL, Kozell LB, Meshul CK, Bunzow JR, Low MJ, Levine MS, Grandy DK: Dopamine D_4 receptor-deficient mice display cortical hyperexcitability. J Neurosci 2001; 21:3756–3763.

23 Wang X, Zhong P, Yan Z: Dopamine D_4 receptors modulate GABAergic signaling in pyramidal neurons of prefrontal cortex. J Neurosci 2002;22:9185–9193.

24 Apud JA, Weinberger DR: Treatment of cognitive deficits associated with schizophrenia: potential role of catechol-O-methyltransferase inhibitors. CNS Drugs 2007;21:535–557.

25 Woodward ND, Jayathilake K, Meltzer HY: COMT va1108/158met genotype, cognitive function, and cognitive improvement with clozapine in schizophrenia. Schizophr Res 2007;90:86–96.

26 Vale S: Current management of the cognitive dysfunction in Parkinson's disease: how far have we come? Exp Biol Med (Maywood) 2008;233:941–951.

27 Varty GB, Bakshi VP, Geyer MA: M100907, a serotonin $5-HT_{2A}$ receptor antagonist and putative antipsychotic, blocks dizocilpine-induced prepulse inhibition deficits in Sprague-Dawley and Wistar rats. Neuropsychopharmacology 1999;20:311–321.

28 Alex KD, Pehek EA: Pharmacologic mechanisms of serotonergic regulation of dopamine neurotransmission. Pharmacol Ther 2007;113:296–320.

29 Poyurovsky M, Koren D, Gonopolsky I, Schneidman M, Fuchs C, Weizman A, Weizman R: Effect of the $5-HT_2$ antagonist mianserin on cognitive dysfunction in chronic schizophrenia patients: an add-on, double-blind placebo-controlled study. Eur Neuropsychopharmacol 2003;13:123–128.

30 Roth BL, Hanizavareh SM, Blum AE: Serotonin receptors represent highly favorable molecular targets for cognitive enhancement in schizophrenia and other disorders. Psychopharmacology (Berl) 2004;174:17–24.

31 Bowen DM, Francis PT, Chessell IP, Webster MT: Neurotransmission–the link integrating Alzheimer research? Trends Neurosci 1994;17:149–150.

32 Ichikawa J, Ishii H, Bonaccorso S, Fowler WL, O'Laughlin IA, Meltzer HY: $5-HT_{2A}$ and D_2 receptor blockade increases cortical DA release via $5-HT_{1A}$ receptor activation: a possible mechanism of atypical antipsychotic-induced cortical dopamine release. J Neurochem 2001;76:1521–1531.

33 Yuen EY, Jiang Q, Chen P, Gu Z, Feng J, Yan Z: Serotonin 5-HT$_{1A}$ receptors regulate NMDA receptor channels through a microtubule-dependent mechanism. J Neurosci 2005;25:5488–5501.

34 Meltzer HY, Sumiyoshi T: Does stimulation of 5-HT$_{1A}$ receptors improve cognition in schizophrenia? Behav Brain Res 2008;195:98–102.

35 Terry AV Jr, Buccafusco JJ, Wilson C: Cognitive dysfunction in neuropsychiatric disorders: selected serotonin receptor subtypes as therapeutic targets. Behav Brain Res 2008;195:30–38.

36 Foley AG, Murphy KJ, Hirst WD, Gallagher HC, Hagan JJ, Upton N, Walsh FS, Regan CM: The 5-HT$_6$ receptor antagonist SB-271046 reverses scopolamine-disrupted consolidation of a passive avoidance task and ameliorates spatial task deficits in aged rats. Neuropsychopharmacology 2004;29:93–100.

37 Manuel-Apolinar L, Meneses A: 8-OH-DPAT facilitated memory consolidation and increased hippocampal and cortical cAMP production. Behav Brain Res 2004;148:179–184.

38 Ji XH, Ji JZ, Zhang H, Li BM: Stimulation of α2-adrenoceptors suppresses excitatory synaptic transmission in the medial prefrontal cortex of rat. Neuropsychopharmacology 2008;33:2263–2271.

39 Fields RB, Van Kammen DP, Peters JL, Rosen J, Van Kammen WB, Nugent A, Stipetic M, Linnoila M: Clonidine improves memory function in schizophrenia independently from change in psychosis: preliminary findings. Schizophr Res 1988;1:417–423.

40 Friedman JI, Adler DN, Temporini HD, Kemether E, Harvey PD, White L, Parrella M, Davis KL: Guanfacine treatment of cognitive impairment in schizophrenia. Neuropsychopharmacology 2001;25:402–409.

41 Gobert A, Rivet JM, Audinot V, Newman-Tancredi A, Cistarelli L, Millan MJ: Simultaneous quantification of serotonin, dopamine and noradrenaline levels in single frontal cortex dialysates of freely-moving rats reveals a complex pattern of reciprocal auto- and heteroreceptor-mediated control of release. Neuroscience 1998;84:413–429.

42 Friedman JI: Cholinergic targets for cognitive enhancement in schizophrenia: focus on cholinesterase inhibitors and muscarinic agonists. Psychopharmacology (Berl) 2004;174:45–53.

43 Freedman R, Hall M, Adler LE, Leonard S: Evidence in postmortem brain tissue for decreased numbers of hippocampal nicotinic receptors in schizophrenia. Biol Psychiatry 1995;38:22–33.

44 Dean B, McLeod M, Keriakous D, McKenzie J, Scarr E: Decreased muscarinic1 receptors in the dorsolateral prefrontal cortex of subjects with schizophrenia. Mol Psychiatry 2002;7:1083–1091.

45 Chouinard S, Sepehry AA, Stip E: Oral cholinesterase inhibitor add-on therapy for cognitive enhancement in schizophrenia: a quantitative systematic review, part I. Clin Neuropharmacol 2007;30:169–182.

46 Stip E, Sepehry AA, Chouinard S: Add-on therapy with acetylcholinesterase inhibitors for memory dysfunction in schizophrenia: a systematic quantitative review, part 2. Clin Neuropharmacol 2007;30:218–229.

47 Buchanan RW, Conley RR, Dickinson D, Ball MP, Feldman S, Gold JM, McMahon RP: Galantamine for the treatment of cognitive impairments in people with schizophrenia. Am J Psychiatry 2008;165:82–89.

48 Lee SW, Lee JG, Lee BJ, Kim YH: A 12-week, double-blind, placebo-controlled trial of galantamine adjunctive treatment to conventional antipsychotics for the cognitive impairments in chronic schizophrenia. Int Clin Psychopharmacol 2007;22:63–68.

49 Dyer MA, Freudenreich O, Culhane MA, Pachas GN, Deckersbach T, Murphy E, Goff DC, Evins AE: High-dose galantamine augmentation inferior to placebo on attention, inhibitory control and working memory performance in nonsmokers with schizophrenia. Schizophr Res 2008;102:88–95.

50 Martin LF, Freedman R: Schizophrenia and the α7 nicotinic receptor. Int Rev Neurobiol 2007;78:225–246.

51 Benwell ME, Balfour DJ, Birrell CE: Desensitization of the nicotine-induced mesolimbic dopamine responses during constant infusion with nicotine. Br J Pharmacol 1995;114:454–460.

52 Simosky JK, Stevens KE, Freeman R: Nicotinic agonists and psychosis. Curr Drug Targets CNS Neurol Disord 2002;1:149–162.

53 Sellin AK, Shad M, Tamminga C: Muscarinic agonists for the treatment of cognition in schizophrenia. CNS Spectr 2008;13:985–996.

54 Raedler TJ, Bymaster FP, Tandon R, Copolov D, Dean B: Towards a muscarinic hypothesis of schizophrenia. Mol Psychiatry 2007;12:232–246.

55 Mirza NR, Peters D, Sparks RG: Xamomeline and the antipsychotic potential of muscarinic receptor subtype selective agonists. CNS Drug Rev 2003;9:159–186.

56 Javitt DC: Glutamate as a therapeutic target in psychiatric disorders. Mol Psychiatry 2004;9:984–997, 979.

57 Buchanan RW, Javitt DC, Marder SR, Schooler NR, Gold JM, McMahon RP, Heresco-Levy U, Carpenter WT: The Cognitive and Negative Symptoms in Schizophrenia Trial (CONSIST): the efficacy of glutamatergic agents for negative symptoms and cognitive impairments. Am J Psychiatry 2007;164:1593–1602.

58 Shim SS, Hammonds MD, Kee BS: Potentiation of the NMDA receptor in the treatment of schizophrenia: focused on the glycine site. Eur Arch Psychiatry Clin Neurosci 2008;258:16–27.

59 Tsai G, Lane HY, Yang P, Chong MY, Lange N: Glycine transporter I inhibitor, N-methylglycine (sarcosine) added to antipsychotics for the treatment of schizophrenia. Biol Psychiatry 2004;55:452–456.

60 Lane HY, Chang YC, Liu YC, Chiu CC, Tasi GE: Sarcosine or D-serine add-on treatment for acute exacerbation of schizophrenia: a randomized, double-blind, placebo-controlled study. Arch Gen Psychiatry 2005;62:1196–1204.

61 Lane HY, Huang CL, Wu PL, Liu YC, Chang YC, Lin PY, Chen PW, Tsai G: Glycine transporter I inhibitor, N-methylglycine (sarcosine), added to clozapine for the treatment of schizophrenia. Biol Psychiatry 2006; 60:645–649.

62 Goff DC, Lamberti JS, Leon AC, Green MF, Miller AL, Patel J, Manschreck T, Freudenreich O, Johnson SA: A placebo-controlled add-on trial of the ampakine, CX516, for cognitive deficits in schizophrenia. Neuropsychopharmacology 2008;33:465–472.

63 Lewis DA, Cho RY, Carter CS, Eklund K, Forster S, Kelly MA, Montrose D: Subunit-selective modulation of GABA type A receptor neurotransmission and cognition in schizophrenia. Am J Psychiatry 2008;165:1585–1593, erratum in Am J Psychiatry 2009;166:120.

Priv.-Doz. Dr. Alex Hofer
Medical University Innsbruck
Department of Psychiatry and Psychotherapy, Biological Psychiatry Division
6020 Innsbruck (Austria)
Tel. +43 512 504 23669, Fax +43 512 504 25267, E-Mail a.hofer@i-med.ac.at

Roder V, Medalia A (eds): Neurocognition and Social Cognition in Schizophrenia Patients. Basic Concepts and Treatment. Key Issues Ment Health. Basel, Karger, 2010, vol 177, pp 158–172

7

Motivational Enhancements in Schizophrenia

Alice Medalia · Jimmy Choi

Department of Psychiatry, Columbia University College of Physicians and Surgeons, New York, N.Y., USA

Abstract

This chapter reviews the role of motivation in learning outcomes, a relevant topic for cognitive remediation programs which seek to enhance learning of neuropsychological skills. The literature indicates that people with schizophrenia who participate in cognitive remediation are more likely to benefit from the programs if they are intrinsically motivated to work on the tasks to improve their cognition. This intrinsic motivation refers to the motivation to attend the program because improved cognition is valued as a goal in and of itself. Since participants are not always intrinsically motivated when they enroll in cognitive remediation programs, it is important for clinicians to know that intrinsic motivation can be manipulated by applying certain instructional techniques and that when these techniques are used, the learning outcomes are increased. There is now evidence that people with schizophrenia respond to some of the same instructional techniques known to enhance intrinsic motivation in healthy students. The adaptable nature of intrinsic motivational processes in schizophrenia provides a platform from which to design effective cognitive remediation programs to enhance not only cognition but also functional outcome.

Cognitive remediation programs have enjoyed success in improving the neuropsychological deficits so evident in schizophrenia. Recent reviews of randomized, controlled trials of cognitive training reveal that on average, studies show moderate effect size improvements on a variety of neurocognitive measures [1, 2]. Training on cognitive exercises elevated cognitive performance to a level consistent with that of healthy controls, produced generalization of improvement to other neurocognitive tasks [3] with durable cognitive improvements lasting up to 2 years [4]. Thus, cognitive rehabilitation has surfaced as a behavioral treatment modality for schizophrenia that is distinct from other psychosocial treatments for psychosis in that it directly targets the neurocognitive impairment that frequently accompanies the illness.

Many components play a significant role in the successful rehabilitation of cognitive deficits in schizophrenia. For example, most recent empirical research suggests that integrating cognitive remediation with other methods of psychiatric rehabilitation (supported employment, social skills training, etc.) may be more effective than individual approaches in achieving overall psychiatric rehabilitation [1]. Cognitive ability [5], instructional techniques [6] and therapist qualification are other factors that can impact the treatment outcome [7]. It is also recognized that there is an interplay between neurocognitive recovery and the psychological states which influence the actual learning process [8]. One such mechanism beginning to receive more empirical examination is the role of *motivation* and its associated derivatives in cognitive recovery and overall psychiatric rehabilitation.

Motivation has long been recognized as a key predictor of learning in students enrolled in formal education programs. In healthy normals, motivation is fundamental to persistence and adherence to tasks that involve complex information processing or creativity [9]. Increasingly there is appreciation of the role motivation plays in the learning process that takes place when people with schizophrenia participate in cognitive remediation. Motivated patients are more likely to complete the tasks within a specified therapeutic time period rather than become disengaged and at risk for attrition and/or insufficient treatment intensity [10]. Furthermore, motivated patients seem to benefit more from the treatment – that is they make greater cognitive improvement [7]. Given the role that motivation plays in the treatment outcome, it is important to consider how best to teach neurocognitive skills to people whose illness causes a lack of motivation and insight, and for all intents and purposes, a profound learning disability that limits the ability to generalize acquired information into functional skills.

Motivation and Learning

Motivation literally means to be moved to do something and refers to the processes whereby goal-directed activities are instigated and sustained. Without motivation a person is passive, apathetic and even inert and unresponsive. In the psychotherapeutic context, motivation is associated with engagement in treatment, persistence of adaptive behaviors, attendance at sessions, willingness to do tasks, activity level, initiative, learning, treatment compliance and extent of reliance on others.

In the context of learning situations, motivation is associated with greater learning and more persistence on tasks. People with schizophrenia often demonstrate decreased motivation to participate in learning activities. Even when they indicate that learning is a valued goal, they may not demonstrate the behaviors that facilitate learning. They may miss sessions or forget assignments. This likely occurs not because they do not want to learn but because of a negative interaction between a physiologically based deficit in motivation and social contextual determinants of motivation. For example, the physiologically based decrease in motivation may influence whether patients in fact initiate and then sustain learning behaviors. When patients fail to initiate behavior even toward goals perceived as worthy, they in turn fail to develop competencies to meet their learning goals. Then, when faced with a new learning situation (like cognitive rehabilitation), the patient anticipates failure on the tasks, which further deflates the motivation to improve cognition. Given this destructive vicious circle, it is crucial to consider the factors that serve as determinants of motivation so that appropriate steps can be taken to intervene and stop the vicious circle of withdrawal from learning activities.

Determinants of Motivation

Motivation can be thought of as the product of a complex interaction of physiological and social contextual determinants. The physiological determinants have become a focus of investigation relatively recently, and neuroscientists are beginning to understand how the absence of the neurotransmitter dopamine can lower drive- and goal-directed behavior [11]. Deficits in dopamine function can lead to disruptions in the drive to attain rewards in task learning, even if the reward is perceived as pleasurable and desirable. This is especially relevant given the predominant view of dopaminergic disturbances in the pathophysiology of schizophrenia. Medication is variably successful at targeting avolition, a negative symptom state that can sometimes be quite severe. Thus, it is all the more crucial to consider the social contextual factors that serve as determinants of motivation. The social contextual determinants of motivation have been and continue to be extensively studied, and there is lively debate about the factors in the environment that affect motivation. Ultimately physiological and social contextual variables intertwine to affect the constitutional, trait-like motivational style as well as the situational motivational responses of an individual.

When considering motivation in a learning situation like cognitive remediation, it can be useful to take into account not only the amount or level of motivation but also the processes that lead one to want to learn and then actually engage in learning. Theories of motivation to learn often cite the role of expectancies, values and goal orientation in the learning process. Wigfield and Eccles [12], two leading researchers in the field of motivation, suggest that in fact one could understand the motivation to learn by asking 3 questions. Do I *expect* success in the learning task? Do I *value* the task? *Why* do I want to do the task? It is deceptively simple to consider that motivation could be accounted for by posing these 3 questions; in fact research has articulated complex mechanisms – that lead to expectations of success and explain how and why people value tasks – and the nature of the goal orientation that determines why someone wants to learn. In the following sections we will first review some of this literature and then also consider how the findings may be applicable in the cognitive remediation setting.

Do I Expect Success in the Learning Task?

Expectations of success are related to the perception of one's ability (self-efficacy) and of the difficulty of the task [13]. In the setting of cognitive remediation, the patients who have grown to doubt their ability after experiencing failure at school or work may be reluctant to engage in the treatment. Schizophrenia has an insidious onset and there is often a subtle deterioration in cognitive skills that can lead to academic decline. Students who once had facility for learning may start to experience difficulty and then slowly begin to doubt their ability to succeed in learning tasks. It is not at all uncommon to have patients come into cognitive remediation with a mind-set that predicts failure. According to motivational theory, that expectation of failure will affect the motivation to participate in treatment and to do the tasks [12, 13].

Self-efficacy or perceived competency at learning affects the choice of learning tasks, effort on tasks, persistence at learning exercises and achievement [14]. When people think they will be good at a task, they are more willing to persist at it and typically achieve a higher level. Those who anticipate being competent choose harder tasks and are more willing to try new ones. They exert more effort because they think they will succeed. There is considerable research demonstrating the role of perceived competency in healthy normals and now data are showing that when people have schizophrenia, there is similarly a large role for perceived competency in learning outcomes [15].

We recently examined the degree to which perceptions of self-competency for a difficult cognitive task contributed to the amount of learning in adults with schizophrenia. In this study [8], we directly compared one learning method that incorporated intrinsically motivating strategies known to enhance learning in healthy normal adolescents [16] against another method that carefully manipulated out the motivational variables in the same learning program. Arithmetic provided a gauge of direct domain-specific learning so that we could quantify the degree of material absorption from a specific training program. The lessons were taught through parallel computer-based arithmetic learning programs with and without the motivational embellishments. As expected and consistent with findings in healthy controls [17], people with schizophrenia who received the arithmetic lessons embedded in a motivational teaching paradigm demonstrated greater acquisition of arithmetic skills, higher levels of intrinsic motivation for the task, and greater feelings of self-efficacy and achievement to tackle the challenging lessons. Importantly, higher perceived competency even prior to training predicted greater improvement in arithmetic scores for people in either training program, even after variance attributable to cognition, perceptions of treatment autonomy and intrinsic motivation had been accounted for. These findings support the notion that these constructs are operative in schizophrenia. Instructional techniques that enhanced perceptions of self-competency also improved learning. Similarly to the nonpsychiatric population, people with schizophrenia must believe their actions can produce the outcomes they desire (self-competency), or else they may have little incentive or motivation to take on challenging cognitive tasks in remediation programs.

Why Do People Expect Success in Learning Tasks?
Expectations of success in learning are related to multiple variables. The anticipation of competency on a learning task is linked to the perception of its difficulty. Tasks that immediately appear complicated will generate a negative expectation, while tasks that can be more easily grasped will influence a positive expectation of learning success. Past performance, role models, the persuasiveness of feedback on performance, physiological indicators, goal properties of the task and beliefs about the malleability of intelligence are other factors that impact the expectation of success in learning tasks [12–14, 18].

Dweck's implicit personality theory [18] informs us that motivation for success is influenced both by a person's goal orientation and their cognitive appraisal of action outcomes. Goal orientation can be dichotomized into performance goals, where competence is measured relative to others, or mastery goals, where competence is assessed relative to task mastery. In a performance goal orientation, the focus of task success is on the reaction of other people (demonstrating competency) and fear of failure. In task mastery or otherwise called 'learning goal orientation', the focus is on the innate improvement of one's own competence irrespective of other people's reactions. Performance goals are associated with the belief that intelligence is fixed and the desire to avoid an exhibition of deficiency. Failure on the task is attributed to a lack of ability and makes the individual vulnerable to feelings of helplessness and negative assessments regarding performance, ultimately leading to task avoidance. In contrast, a learning goal orientation is associated with the view that intelligence is malleable and a belief that expending effort will improve ability.

People with a learning goal orientation are more amendable to remediation, since they believe that effort can enhance the likelihood of success in a task. According to Dweck's theory, interventions that encourage a learning goal orientation and belief that intelligence is malleable should assist people with schizophrenia to subscribe to cognitive remediation as a valuable activity. For example, psychoeducation about cognition in schizophrenia and demonstration of task improvement may illustrate the concept that cognition is malleable. Once patients understand that cognition can change and that they control the variation by applying effort, they may more readily engage in the learning process. When patients encounter a challenging task (e.g. cognitive training) and form their expectations for success, a learning goal orientation is likely to lead to greater intrinsic motivation, receptiveness to remediation programs and engagement in learning sessions.

Expectations of success are also guided by past performance and physiological reactions to the task. Repeated failures at a task tend to lower self-efficacy and implant doubt about learning capability, so methods to titrate difficulty are paramount to instilling motivation for achievement (see errorless learning in this chapter). Physiological reactions such as sweating or increased heart rate are biofeedback markers of excess arousal and anxiety and interpreted as incompetency in the face of a task, so environmental and therapeutic milieus which encourage a calm but stimulating state may promote high perceptions of aptitude and optimize the learning experience.

Expectation of Success in Learning: Implications for Practice
The research on perceived competency to learn has implications for cognitive remediation and suggests that if clinicians consider techniques to enhance self-efficacy in the learning situation, they may be able to maximize the therapeutic outcomes. This can be difficult, especially since many patients may enter into the programs with low perceived self-competence for learning. One technique which has received positive attention is errorless learning.

Errorless learning is based on promoting the desired response through a sequence of incremental changes in task difficulty level. This theoretically and empirically driven model of implicit learning was designed to compensate for impairments in cognition that limit initial learning skill acquisition. Basic and clinical laboratory studies have shown that learning occurring in the absence of errors is stronger and more durable than the traditional trial-and-error alternative. To avoid excessive errors, training commences at a carefully set point where there is an expectation for success and then gradually advances through progressively more difficult exercises. Importantly, successful performance is maintained at each difficulty level because of the diminutive increments in task demand, thus, sustaining a relatively positive experience in contrast to incessant feedback on repeated mistakes.

Errorless learning was first used as a method of operational conditioning that eliminated or minimized responding to incorrect behavioral choices in developmentally delayed children. The strategy was adapted for a number of neurologic and neuropsychiatric impairments, including memory and language rehabilitation for head injury, aphasia, dementia and schizophrenia [19]. More recently, Kern et al. [20] introduced the framework of errorless learning to skills training programs for people with schizophrenia and found that repetitive, successful practice within the context of a rich schedule of positive reinforcement promoted self-efficacy and generalization of learned skills to different social and work situations.

Another technique that may enhance the perceived self-competency to learn is the careful titration of the goal properties of the tasks [21]. Tasks which have distal and vague goals may be perceived as too difficult, while those with proximal, clearly defined aims are likely to be seen as more manageable. For example, a sorting task which requires categorization of 9 objects along 2 known vectors (e.g. shape and color) has a more proximal and well-defined goal than a sorting task which involves categorization of 15 items along 3 vectors 'to be determined' (e.g. the patient must deduce from feedback that the vectors are shape, color and size). People with a limited working memory would have difficulty keeping multiple goal features in mind, and therefore could easily disengage from the task because it is perceived as too cognitively challenging, and failure at the task is anticipated. Giving patients tasks with goal properties that are appropriate to their cognitive capacity and psychological tolerance for failure can enhance the motivation to do the task.

The feedback that a patient receives while learning can also impact self-efficacy [21]. Positive feedback can be an effective means to motivate a person who is experiencing difficulty on a demanding task, but it can demotivate if it is not credible [14]. For example, an instructor who walks around the room and tells everybody 'good job' regardless of whether someone is doing well, is not providing any consequential validation for performance or effort. However, an instructor who reinforces specific performance and effort by providing a credible statement such as 'I saw how you did that task and know that you can do this' offers more substantiation to the learner and, in turn, generates greater expectations of success. Credible feedback is specific and well timed, and it is most effective when corroborated by actual performance [17]. Increased motivation and expectations will be confirmed if the learner succeeds in the task, but the impact will be fleeting if the learner attempts the task and performs poorly.

There are many types of feedback, such as performance, corrective, attributional and strategy feedback [14]. Some forms can come from self-monitoring, while others may be external, from the clinician. *Attributional feedback*, which is a persuasive source of self-efficacy information, links success with effort or ability. A statement about effort – 'You did that right, you're really working hard' – supports the patients' perceptions of their progress, sustains motivation and increases self-efficacy. The timing of feedback is also important. When patients first start to work on an exercise, effort feedback is more credible than ability feedback, but as they acquire skills the task becomes easier, so ability feedback gains credibility. *Performance feedback* provides information about progress in learning and should raise motivation and learning. Many software activities are designed to provide performance feedback. In addition, the patients can be asked to engage in performance tracking which prompts them to be continually self-aware of their ongoing performance and cognitive activity level. This awareness encourages metacognition and ultimately a more accurate synchrony between their goals and abilities. Participants with psychosis who are continually made self-aware of their performance and cognitive activity level seem to engage in a self-monitoring process that has been shown to improve the outcome in cognitive remediation [22, 23]. Methods to engage participants by monitoring their own performance, either by making notes on paper or verbally describing their thought processes, seem to provide an effective information processing feedback loop that allows participants to steadily progress and visualize the rewards by actually seeing their progress from one session to another.

Expectations of success in cognitive tasks are also sensitive to the effects of modeling. In modeling, self-efficacy is impacted by vicarious learning experiences as opposed to active learning experiences. Students that anticipate they will be successful because they have observed someone they can emulate or identify with successfully perform a task. According to Bandura's social cognitive theory [24], modeling can instill self-efficacy in the learner when the learner believes that the model is demonstrating a valuable skill and also that the model is similar to the learner in skill capacity (i.e. peer). Interestingly, authority or expert models do not instill the same sense of self-efficacy because they are seen as so dissimilar. In much the same manner, participants in cognitive remediation programs may not undergo such an ego-building vicarious learning experience if competent clinicians or therapists continually demonstrate the skill. Rather, patients may be more motivated to attend to models and retain the lesson content if they observe their fellow peers succeeding in a demanding task and developing new skills. For this reason it can be helpful to conduct cognitive remediation in a group setting and to incorporate peer leadership into the program. Even if patients are working independently on tasks, if they share the learning experience in a room with others who are also engaged in learning, they experience a positive vicarious learning atmosphere. Maybe the person next to them has a big smile because she successfully completed the task, maybe they see someone try a new activity and seem pleased, maybe they hear someone sound happy that they got the right answer. All these experiences shape the perception that 'if they can learn, so can I'. The other members in the group serve as 'coping models' [17], who initially display difficulties but through persistence and effort gradually improve their performance and eventually succeed. Peer leaders offer another source of modeling because they explain and demonstrate skills and convey to patients that they too can be successful if they perform the same actions.

Do I Value the Task?

People are more likely to engage in a learning activity if they perceive its value [25]. This is particularly true for adults, who are less willing than children to do something simply because they have been told to. The value of a learning activity can come from the interest it generates, or because it has perceived utility vis-à-vis reaching one's goals, or as it helps one attain a future or desired self. Cost is a fourth dimension that is applied to the assessment of the value of a task. It allows the weighing of the comparative merits of investing time and energy in different tasks and assumes a finite expenditure of energy and resources.

People who are unclear about their goals and the kind of person they want to be may be particularly drawn by the interest value of a task. Interest value refers to how enjoyable the task is. In the setting of cognitive remediation, this is the enjoyment derived from performing a cognitive enhancing task. Since people vary in what they perceive as interesting and enjoyable, not all tasks will be viewed similarly by patients. However, some tasks tend to be more commonly referred to as dull and boring than others. When tasks lack interest value, and the patient cannot readily see the utility or attainment value, motivation may be jeopardized.

On the other hand, if a person sees the utility of doing a task, that is they can relate performance of the activity to their short- and long-range goals, then it may not be as necessary for the task to be enjoyable and fun to perform [25]. Then the gratification of doing the task comes from the perceived link between performance and goal attainment. Speculatively, one reason that cognitive remediation programs may be more effective when combined with psychiatric rehabilitation programs is that the utility value of the cognitive remediation program is more evident. Patients may be more motivated to participate and learn because the cognitive exercises are seen as having utility for getting back to work, going to school or living independently. One way to assist patients to appreciate the utility value of a cognitive task is to explicitly link performance on it to achievement of their goals. This can be done individually, by discussing the task with the patient, or it can be done in groups that bridge cognitive remediation to daily life. A number of cognitive remediation programs utilize bridging discussions, and these not only enhance metacognition but may serve to enhance motivation by highlighting the utility value of participating in treatment.

Attainment value differs from interest and utility value because the emphasis is on whether engaging in the activity can increase the likelihood of obtaining a desired future self or avoiding an undesired future self [25]. In learning settings, the impact of attainment value is evident when someone says: 'My father has a great memory; I would like to be like him', or 'I don't want to be like those people who just think all the time; I don't need this'. When cognitive remediation is conducted in groups and peer leaders are used, attainment value can be an operative determinant of someone's motivation to participate and learn. Seeing a peer patient who is likeable and good at the tasks may motivate others to attain good cognitive functioning.

Cost is the fourth consideration that informs the ultimate value of a task. Wigfield and Eccles [25] have highlighted the importance of considering this dimension which refers to the emotional and practical cost of choosing one activity over another. People who choose to partake in cognitive remediation may be limiting their access to another therapy, they may have to juggle family responsibilities or finances, or they may have to consider their overall capacity to take on multiple commitments given the context of an illness that causes one to easily feel overwhelmed. When the costs of participating in cognitive remediation or any therapy are too high, patients may choose not to engage in that activity, even if they value the anticipated outcome of the therapy. On the other hand, not participating may have such a high cost that the patient is impelled toward participation.

Now let us turn our attention to the third reason people are motivated to learn.

Why Do I Want to Do the Task?

According to the self-determination theory, individuals will be most motivated to engage in tasks if they believe they had choice and that they made the decision to do the task, if they think they will be competent at the task and value the accompanying social interactions [9]. When these needs are fulfilled in a learning situation – that is the needs for mastery, personal control and attachment – then people will find learning inherently enjoyable and be motivated to continue participating in the activity. This inherent enjoyment in the task is called intrinsic motivation. Intrinsic motivation, in the context of a learning environment, refers to the desire to engage in a learning activity because it is inherently interesting and engaging. This contrasts with extrinsic motivation, which refers to the motivation to learn because a tangible extrinsic result will occur, for example a prize or money.

Considerable research indicates that in a learning environment, intrinsic motivation is associated with greater learning, higher performance persistence, more creativity, higher self-esteem and sense of well-being, and greater engagement in surroundings [26]. Extrinsic motivators, on the other hand, can decrease the amount of learning that takes place, and educators are thus advised to use them judiciously [27–29].

If one assumes that people with schizophrenia will learn like students without schizophrenia, then in the setting of cognitive remediation, intrinsic motivation should enhance the learning outcomes. This is in fact supported by 2 studies that found dramatic differences in effect size when participants in a cognitive remediation program were divided into high and low intrinsic motivation on the basis of their voluntary, frequent attendance at the program [7]. Participants in community-based cognitive remediation programs have the option to attend or not, and regular attendance can thus be used as a measure of intrinsic motivation. Both studies found large effect sizes on an untrained clerical task of processing speed for the intrinsically motivated group. In contrast, the participants who were not intrinsically motivated achieved a very small effect size on this outcome measure.

The impact of intrinsic motivation is not limited to neuropsychological outcomes. A recent paper clearly illustrates how intrinsic motivation mediates the impact of neurocognition on psychosocial outcome [30]. Nakagami et al. [30] examined the nature of the relationships among neurocognition, intrinsic motivation and psychosocial functioning in 120 schizophrenia patients enrolled in outpatient psychosocial rehabilitation. They found that intrinsic motivation significantly mediated the link between neurocognition and psychosocial functioning, but interestingly, neurocognition did not influence the relationship between intrinsic motivation and psychosocial functioning. The denoted strength of the relationship between intrinsic motivation and both neurocognition and psychosocial functioning suggests that intrinsic motivation promotes neurocognitive improvement and that intrinsic motivation is also vital to strategies for improving functional levels for individuals with schizophrenia.

Given the role of intrinsic motivation in learning, it becomes important to consider the social contextual variables that can enhance or diminish it. This understanding can then be used to inform the instructional techniques used in a cognitive remediation program, which should in turn enhance the effectiveness of the treatment and improve the ability to disseminate it to community settings where extrinsic motivators like subject reimbursement are not operative.

Determinants of Intrinsic Motivation to Learn

In an educational setting, the social contextual variables that impact intrinsic motivation to learn are manifested as interpersonal context, instructional techniques and the general learning environment. Interpersonal context refers to the relationship between teacher and student, as well as between students. The nature of these interpersonal contexts has been shown to affect the attainment of learning goals. Controlling social contexts that pressure people through the use of incentives, deadlines and authoritarian commentary reduce a sense of autonomy, self-determination and motivation [27]. Moreover, controlling social contexts results in greater passivity, decreased persistence in learning activities and poorer learning. Conversely, social contexts that minimize the salience of external incentives, avoid controlling language and acknowledge the learner's individuality are more likely to enhance the intrinsic motivation, test performance, amount of learning and sense of well-being.

These principles also apply to people with schizophrenia, and arguably to all patients enrolled in rehabilitation programs [31]. Indeed from a psychiatric rehabilitation perspective, the relationship between the cognitive remediation therapist and patient is a key factor in responsiveness to treatment, and creating an autonomy-supportive environment would be consistent with the empirically based principles that ground the psychiatric rehabilitation field. Patients in psychiatric rehabilitation programs who are involved in setting their own goals have greater chances of achieving their goals, a finding that highlights the merits of autonomy-supportive treatment environments.

In cognitive remediation programs, autonomy-supportive environments are learning environments where the instructor supports and guides the student's interests and emerging desire to learn. The role of the clinician is not simply to oversee the completion of a prescribed generic template of tasks, say a particular software program given to everyone, but to observe, assess and guide in the use of exercises specific to the individual's needs [21]. There is emerging empirical evidence that intrinsic motivation to learn is enhanced in an autonomy-supportive cognitive remediation environment, where people with schizophrenia are allowed to exercise some control over their learning experience, where the value of the activity is evident and opportunities for demonstrating competency exist [8].

Instructional techniques are another social contextual determinant of intrinsic motivation to learn. There are a number of instructional variables that enhance intrinsic motivation such as personalization, choice and contextualization [12], which can be embedded into a specific activity or into the overall treatment plan. Contextualization means that rather than presenting material in the abstract, it is put in a context, whereby the practical utility and link to everyday life activities are made obvious to the client. For example, in attention remediation, a decontextualized focusing task would require the person to press a button every time a yellow circle appears on the otherwise blank computer screen. In contrast, a contextualized focusing task would require the person to assume the role of a train conductor in a task which simulated the experience of responding to a track signal. Personalization refers to the tailoring of a learning activity to coincide with topics of high interest value for the client. For example, if the person likes to travel, he is more likely to enjoy a problem-solving task that has him negotiating the challenges that arise when driving a delivery truck, rather than doing a task which teaches problem solving by requiring identification of like-colored objects among an array of shapes. Personalization also refers to the learner entering into the task as an identifiable and independent agent, for example signing in by name or assuming a role (stock broker, detective or musician) in a task that simulates a real-world activity.

Learner control refers to the provision of choices within the learning activity, in order to foster self-determination. In memory training, this occurs when the client can choose task features like difficulty level or presence of additional auditory cues when doing a visual memory exercise. Learner control can also be provided by structuring the sessions so that the participants have opportunities to choose their learning activity, as opposed to being told what they have to work on. Since there are numerous software activities that effectively target specific cognitive skills, there are many opportunities to provide participants with choice and personalized learning experiences.

While it was initially unclear if people with schizophrenia responded to these same social contextual and instructional variables as students without schizophrenia, research now indicates that they do. In a randomized trial that directly compared instructional techniques, it was possible to determine the impact of motivationally enhancing instruction on learning outcomes [8]. By *contextualizing* the cognitive task into a meaningful game-like context, *personalizing* incidental features of the learning process and providing activity *choices* during the task, adults with schizophrenia acquired more cognitive skill, possessed greater intrinsic motivation for a cognitive task, reported greater feelings of self-competency after treatment and demonstrated better attention resource allocation than patients randomly assigned to a generic instructional condition. This study indicates that people with schizophrenia do indeed have a motivational system which is malleable and responsive to the same social contextual cues reported to enhance intrinsic motivation to learn in normals.

Using Motivational Theory to Enhance Treatment Outcomes

Knowing that people with schizophrenia have a motivational system that is malleable and responsive to social contextual cues has important implications for the design of cognitive remediation programs. It means that in addition to considering the purely cognitive aspect of the program – e.g. what areas of cognition to target

– it is productive to be vigilant about how to conduct the treatment. The structure of the sessions and the exercises themselves, the interactions with the clinician and peers, and the design of the curriculum can impact whether patients stay in treatment and how much they benefit from it. Motivation theory indicates that a program that structures sessions and uses activities that provide opportunities for learner control, an experience of competence and positive relationships will foster intrinsic motivation to learn, which will in turn enhance the learning outcomes.

When patients with psychosis are intrinsically motivated for a difficult treatment, they engage in targeted behaviors because of the interest, enjoyment and satisfaction derived from their engagement in the activity, rather than exclusively due to external rewards such as monetary reinforcement or performance certificates [21]. Furthermore, enhancing motivation for training tends to increase the likelihood patients will complete the tasks within a specified therapeutic time period rather than become disengaged and at risk for attrition and/or insufficient treatment intensity [8]. Consequently, intrinsically motivated behaviors are repeated without extensive external rewards or constraints and, therefore, more likely to be maintained within a treatment setting. This is especially relevant to developing treatments in schizophrenia, since experiences of external reward and reinforcement are diminished in schizophrenia [32, 33]. Therefore, it is pragmatic and empirically prudent to focus efforts on targeting and increasing the patients' innate enjoyment and value they place on the training itself rather than relying on platforms of external reward.

The push for understanding the role of intrinsic motivation to enhance the treatment outcome in schizophrenia does not in any way debase the need for the judicious use of extrinsic motivators. Although there is a sizeable literature to show that extrinsic rewards can diminish the innate interest of a task and thereby externalize the motivation for a task that was initially internally driven, the optimal learning experience may employ an arrangement of both external and internal motivating features. There seems to be a mutually inspiring effect where external rewards such as performance feedback *in conjunction with* inherently interesting tasks stimulates intrinsic motivation in unmotivated learners [34]. Learners sometimes rate a task as more intrinsically motivating if there is also a performance-contingent reward. The synergic benefits of both structures of motivation are especially germane for learners who are faced with tasks that have complex and distal goals. Furthermore, appropriate extrinsic motivators like performance feedback may facilitate the gradual internalization of the value of learning and an internalized experience of control and mastery, particularly for tasks perceived as difficult or lacking in inherent interest.

Conclusion

Cognitive remediation programs seek to improve cognitive functioning so that people with schizophrenia will have improved functional outcomes. Approaches to cognitive remediation will be enhanced if they consider not only the neuroscientific bases for cognitive enhancement but also the role of motivation in cognitive and functional outcomes. This chapter has examined the literature on how motivation impacts the learning outcomes in healthy learners and schizophrenia. Evidence indicates that people with schizophrenia participating in cognitive remediation programs are more likely to benefit from the programs if they are intrinsically motivated to improve their cognition. This intrinsic motivation refers to the motivation to attend the program because improved cognition is valued as a goal in and of itself. Theories of motivation highlight the role of social contextual variables in motivating people to learn and in particular focus on the impact of expectations, values and goal properties on learning outcomes. These theories have guided instructors of healthy normals to structure learning in ways that enhance motivation and learning outcomes. We are now beginning to understand that people with schizophrenia respond to some of the same instructional techniques known to enhance intrinsic motivation in healthy students. This has tremendous implications for structuring cognitive remediation programs. The adaptable nature of intrinsic motivational processes in schizophrenia provides an exciting platform from which to design effective cognitive remediation programs to enhance not only cognition but functional outcome.

References

1 McGurk SR, Twamley EW, Sitzer DI, McHugo GJ, Mueser KT: A meta-analysis of cognitive remediation in schizophrenia. Am J Psychiatry 2007;164: 791–802.

2 Twamley EW, Jeste DV, Bellack AS: A review of cognitive training in schizophrenia. Schizophr Bull 2003;29:359–382.

3 Wykes T, Reeder C, Landau S, Everitt B, Knapp M, Patel A, et al: Cognitive remediation therapy in schizophrenia: randomised controlled trial. Br J Psychiatry 2007;190:421–427.

4 Hogarty GE, Flesher S, Ulrich R, Carter M, Greenwald D, Pogue-Geile M, et al: Cognitive enhancement therapy for schizophrenia: effects of a 2-year randomized trial on cognition and behavior. Arch Gen Psychiatry 2004;61:866–876.

5 Fiszdon JM, Choi J, Bryson GJ, Bell MD: Impact of intellectual status on response to cognitive task training in patients with schizophrenia. Schizophr Res 2006;87:261–269.

6 Krabbendam L, Aleman A: Cognitive rehabilitation in schizophrenia: a quantitative analysis of controlled trials. Psychopharmacology 2003;169:376–382.

7 Medalia A, Richardson R: What predicts a good response to cognitive remediation interventions? Schizophr Bull 2005;31:942–953.

8 Choi J, Medalia A: Intrinsic motivation and learning in a schizophrenia spectrum sample. Schizophr Res, in press.

9 Deci EL, Ryan RM: Facilitating optimal motivation and psychological well-being across life's domains. Can Psychol 2008;49:14–23.

10 Choi J, Medalia A: Factors associated with a positive response to cognitive remediation in a community psychiatric sample. Psychiatr Serv 2005;56:602–604.

11 Berridge KC, et al: Affective neuroscience of pleasure: reward in humans and animals. Psychopharmacology 2008;199:457–480.

12 Wigfield A, Eccles JS: Expectancy-value theory of achievement motivation. Contemp Educ Psychol 2000;25:68–81.

13 Bandura A: Toward a psychology of human agency. Perspect Psychol Sci 2006;1:164–180.

14 Schunk DH, Zimmerman BJ (eds): Motivation and Self-Regulated Learning: Theory, Research, and Applications. Mahwah, Erlbaum Associates Publishers, 2008.

15 Medalia A, Choi J: The role of motivation and engagement in successful cognitive training with schizophrenia patients. Schizophr Bull 2009;35:355.

16 Cordova DI, Lepper MR: Intrinsic motivation and the process of learning: beneficial effects of contextualization, personalization, and choice. J Ed Psychol 1996;88:715–730.

17 Zimmerman BJ, Schunk DH: Self-regulating intellectual processes and outcomes: a social cognitive perspective; in Dai DY, Sternberg RJ (eds): Motivation, Emotion, and Cognition. Integrative Perspectives on Intellectual Functioning and Development. Mahwah, Erlbaum Associates Publishers, 2004, pp 323–349.

18 Dweck CS: Self-theories. Their Role in Motivation, Personality, and Development. Philadelphia, Psychology Press, 1999.

19 Clare L, Jones RS: Errorless learning in the rehabilitation of memory impairment: a critical review. Neuropsychol Rev 2008;18:1–23.

20 Kern RS, Green MF, Mitchell S, Kopelowicz A, Mintz J, Liberman RP: Extensions of errorless learning for social problem-solving deficits in schizophrenia. Am J Psychiatry 2005;162:513–519.

21 Medalia A, Revheim N, Herlands T: Cognitive Remediation for psychological Disorders. Therapist Guide. New York, Oxford University Press, 2009.

22 Wykes T, Newton E, Landau S, Rice C, Thompson N, Frangou S: Cognitive remediation therapy (CRT) for young early onset patients with schizophrenia: an exploratory randomized controlled trial. Schizophr Res 2007;94:221–230.

23 Choi J, Kurtz MM: A comparison of remediation techniques on the Wisconsin Card Sorting Test in schizophrenia. Schizophr Res;2009:107:76–82.

24 Bandura A: Going global with social cognitive theory: from prospect to paydirt; in Donaldson SI: Applied Psychology. New Frontiers and Rewarding Careers. Mahwah, Erlbaum Associates Publishers, 2006, pp 53–79.

25 Wigfield A, Eccles JS (eds): Development of Achievement Motivation. San Diego, Academic Press, 2002.

26 Ryan RM, Deci EL: Self-determination theory and the facilitation of intrinsic motivation, social development, and well-being. Am Psychol 2000;55:68–78.

27 Deci EL, Koestner R, Ryan RM: A meta-analytic review of experiments examining the effects of extrinsic rewards on intrinsic motivation. Psychol Bull 1999;125:627–668.

28 Dweck CS: Motivational processes affecting learning. Am Psychologist 1986;41:1040–1048.

29 Dweck CS, Mangels JA, Good C: Motivational effects on attention, cognition, and performance; in Dai DY, Sternberg RJ (eds): Motivation, Emotion, and Cognition: Integrative Perspectives on Intellectual Functioning and Development. Mahwah, Erlbaum Associates, 2004.

30 Nakagami E, Xie B, Hoe M, Brekke J: Intrinsic motivation, neurocognition, and psychosocial functioning in schizophrenia: testing mediator and moderator effects. Schizophr Res 2008;105:95–104.

31 Anthony WA: Cognitive remediation and psychiatric rehabilitation. J Psychiatr Rehabil 2008;32:87–88.

32 Gold JM, Waltz JA, Prentice KJ, Morris SE, Heerey EA: Reward processing in schizophrenia: a deficit in the representation of value. Schizophr Bull 2008;34:835–847.

33 Barch DM: The relationships among cognition, motivation, and emotion in schizophrenia: how much and how little we know. Schizophr Bull 2005;31:875–881.

34 Hidi S, Harackiewicz J: Motivating the academically unmotivated: a critical issue for the 21st century. Rev Educ Res 2000;70:151.

Alice Medalia, PhD
Columbia University College of Physicians and Surgeons
180 Fort Washington Ave., HP 234
New York, NY 10032 (USA)
Tel. +1 212 305 3747, Fax +1 212 305 4724, E-Mail am2938@columbia.edu

Author Index

Subject Index